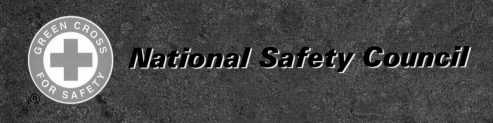

National Safety Council

F1RST AID and CPR

Jones and Bartlett Publishers
Sudbury, Massachusetts

Boston   London   Singapore

Editorial, Sales, and Customer Service Offices

Jones and Bartlett Publishers
40 Tall Pine Drive, Sudbury, MA 01776
Internet: http://www.jbpub.com/nsc/, email: nsc@jbpub.com

Jones and Bartlett Publishers International
Barb House, Barb Mews
London W6 7PA, UK

Library of Congress Cataloging-in-Publication Data
First aid and CPR Standard / National Safety Council
        p.   cm.
    Includes index.
    ISBN 0-7637-0329-X
        1. First aid in illness and injury.   2. CPR (First aid)
    I. National Safety Council.
    RC86.7.F5575   1997
    616.02′52—dc21   96-47633
                                            CIP
First Aid and CPR Essentials:
    ISBN 0-7637-0434-2

Chief Executive Officer: Clayton E. Jones
Emergency Care Editor: Tracy Murphy
Technical Consultant: Alton L. Thygerson
Production Administrator: Anne S. Noonan
Manufacturing Manager: Dana L. Cerrito
Editorial Production Service: Books By Design, Inc.
Illustrations: Rolin Graphics
Interior Stock Photos: Chapter Opener 4 © Bruce Ayres, Tony Stone; Chapter Opener 13 ©
    Wedgewood Custom Medical Publishing; Chapter 16 © Hulton Deutsch, 1994, Picture Network
Typesetting & Pre-press: Pre-Press Company, Inc.
Cover Design: Marshall Henrichs
Cover Photographs: ©Bruce Ayres, Tony Stone; ©Bob Daemmrich, Stock Boston; Steve Ferry,
    P&F Communications
Printing and Binding: Banta Company
Cover Printing: Banta Company

Printed in the United States of America
00 99 98 97   10 9 8 7 6 5 4 3 2

CONTENTS

ABOUT THE NATIONAL SAFETY COUNCIL PROGRAM

Congratulations on selecting the National Safety Council's First Aid and CPR program! You join good company, as the National Safety Council has successfully trained over 2.5 million people worldwide in first aid and cardiopulmonary resuscitation (CPR). The National Safety Council's training network of nearly 10,000 instructors at over 2,500 sites worldwide has established the National Safety Council programs as the standard by which all others are judged.

In setting the standards, the National Safety Council has worked in close cooperation with hundreds of national and international organizations, thousands of corporations, thousands of leading educators, dozens of leading medical organizations, and hundreds of state and local governmental agencies. Their collective input has helped create programs that stand alone in quality. Consider just a few of the National Safety Council's current collaborations:

World's Leading Medical Organizations

The National Safety Council is currently working with both the American Academy of Orthopaedic Surgeons (AAOS) and the Wilderness Medical Society (WMS) to help bring innovative, new training programs to the marketplace. The National Safety Council and the AAOS are developing a new First Responder program and the National Safety Council and the WMS are developing the first-of-its-kind wilderness first aid program.

United States Government

The National Safety Council has developed an innovative computer-based training program for first aid that is currently being used to train United States Postal Service employees.

World's Leading Corporations

Thousands of corporations including Westinghouse, Disney, Exxon, General Motors, Pacific Bell, Ameritech, and U.S. West have selected many of the National Safety Council emergency care programs to train employees.

World's Leading Colleges and Universities

Hundreds of leading colleges and universities are working closely with the National Safety Council to fully develop and implement the Internet Initiative that will establish the National Safety Council as the leading on-line provider of emergency care programs.

Most importantly, in selecting the National Safety Council programs, you can feel confident that the programs are accepted and approved worldwide. You can rely on the National Safety Council. Founded in 1913, the National Safety Council is dedicated to protecting life, promoting health, and reducing accidental death. For more than 80 years, the National Safety Council has been the world's leading authority on safety/injury education.

National Safety Council

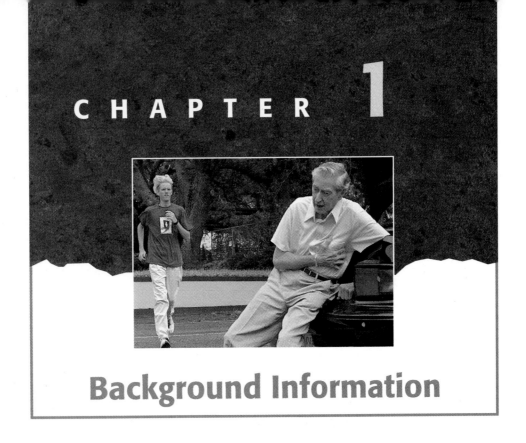

CHAPTER 1

Background Information

Need for First Aid Training

It's better to know first aid and not need it than to need it and not know it. Everyone should be able to perform first aid since most people will eventually find themselves in a situation requiring it, either for another person or for themselves.

A delay of as little as four minutes when a person's heart stops can mean death. Therefore, what a bystander does can mean the difference between life and death. However, most injuries do not require life-saving efforts. During their entire lifetime, most people will see only one or two situations involving life-threatening conditions. While saving lives is important, knowing what to do for less severe injuries demands greater attention and more first aid training.

What Is First Aid?

First aid is the immediate care given to an injured or suddenly ill person. First aid does *not* take the place of proper medical treatment. It consists only of furnishing temporary assistance until competent medical care, if needed, is obtained or until the chance for recovery without medical care is assured. Most injuries and illnesses do not require medical care.

Properly applied, first aid may mean the difference between life and death, rapid recovery and long hospitalization, or temporary disability and permanent injury. First aid involves more than doing things for others; it also includes the things that people can do for themselves.

The ability to recognize a serious medical emergency and knowledge of how to get help may mean the difference between life and death. The problem is that recognition can be delayed because neither the victim nor bystanders know basic symptoms (e.g., a heart attack victim may wait hours after the onset of symptoms before seeking help). Moreover, most people do not know first aid; even if they do, they may panic in an emergency.

Legal Considerations

Legal and ethical issues concern all first aiders.

Consent

Before giving first aid, a first aider must gain consent from a victim. Touching another person without his or her permission or consent is unlawful (known as battery) and could be grounds for a lawsuit. Likewise, giving first aid without the victim's consent is unlawful.

Expressed Consent

Consent must be obtained from every conscious, mentally competent (i.e., able to make a rational decision) adult (i.e., a person of legal age). Tell the victim your name and that you have first aid training and explain what you will be doing. Permission from the victim may be expressed either verbally or with a nod of the head.

Implied Consent

Implied consent involves an unconscious victim and a life-threatening condition. It is assumed or implied that an unresponsive victim would consent to lifesaving interventions. Consent also is implied when the first aider begins care and the victim does not resist.

When life-threatening situations threaten a child, and the parent or legal guardian is not available for consent, first aid should be given based on implied consent. Do not withhold first aid from a minor just to obtain parental or guardian permission.

Abandonment

Abandonment means terminating the care of a victim without ensuring continued care at the same level or higher. Once you have responded to an emergency, you must not leave a victim who needs continuing first aid until another competent and trained person takes responsibility for the victim.

Negligence

Negligence means deviating from accepted standards of care that results in further injury to the victim. Factors involved in negligence include

1. duty to act
2. breach of duty (substandard care)
3. injury and damages inflicted

Duty to Act

No one is required to render first aid when no legal duty exists. Duty to act may occur in the following situations:

- *When employment requires it.* If your employer designates you as responsible for rendering first aid to meet OSHA (Occupational Safety and Health Administration) requirements and you are called to an accident scene, you have a duty to act. Other examples of occupations involving the giving of first aid include law enforcement officers, park rangers, athletic trainers, lifeguards, and teachers, all of whose job descriptions designate them to give first aid.
- *When a preexisting responsibility exists.* You may have a preexisting relationship with other persons that demands you be responsible for them, which means you must give first aid should they need it. Examples include a parent for a child, a driver for a passenger.

Duty to act means following guidelines for standards of care. Standards of care ensure quality care and protection for injured or suddenly ill victims.

Breach of Duty

Generally, a first aider breaches (i.e., "breaks") his or her duty to a victim by failing to provide the type of care that would be provided by a person having the same or similar training. There are two ways to breach one's duty: acts of omission and acts of commission. An *act of omission* is the failure to do what a reasonably prudent person with the same or similar training would do in the same or similar circumstances. An *act of commission* is doing something that a reasonably prudent person would *not* do under the same or similar circumstances. Forgetting to put on a dressing is an act of omission; cutting a snakebite site is an act of commission.

Injury and Damages Inflicted

Other than physical damage, injury and damage can include physical pain and suffering, mental anguish, medical expenses, and sometimes loss of earnings and earning capacity.

Good Samaritan Laws

Laws, known as Good Samaritan laws, encourage people to assist others in distress by granting them immunity against lawsuits. While the laws vary from state to state, Good Samaritan immunity generally applies only when the rescuer is (1) acting during an emergency, (2) acting in good faith, which means he or she has good intentions, (3) acting without compensation, and (4) not guilty of any malicious misconduct or gross negligence toward the victim (deviating from all rational first aid guidelines).

Many legal experts believe that the main effect of Good Samaritan legislation has been to create a false sense of security in the minds of rescuers who erroneously believe that the law protects them from lawsuits regardless of their actions. Good Samaritan laws should not be looked on as a substitute for competent first aid or for keeping within the scope of your training.

While Good Samaritan laws primarily cover medical personnel, several states have expanded them to include laypersons serving as first aiders.

Fear of lawsuits has made some people wary of getting involved in emergency situations. First aiders, however, are rarely sued; for those who are, the courts usually rule in their favor.

Background Information

Directions: Circle Yes if you agree with the statement, and circle No if you disagree.

Yes   No   1. In most locations an ambulance can arrive within minutes. This quick response means that most people do not need to learn to perform first aid.

Yes   No   2. Correct first aid can mean the difference between life and death.

Yes   No   3. Most injuries do no require life-saving first aid efforts.

Yes   No   4. Call for an ambulance and/or seek medical care for all injured victims.

Yes   No   5. In most situations before giving first aid, the victim must give you consent (permission).

Yes   No   6. If you ask a victim if you can help, and she says "No," you can ignore her and proceed giving first aid whether she likes it or not.

Yes   No   7. Employers can designate people as first aiders. This means that they must give first aid to injured employees while on the job.

Yes   No   8. First aiders helping injured victims are often sued.

Yes   No   9. Good Samaritan laws protect first aiders (non-medical personnel) in all states.

Scenario: You are driving slowly looking for a house number in an unfamiliar residential area. You are attempting to deliver an important package to a customer. You see an elderly woman lying at the bottom of porch stairs outside of a house. You see no one else in the neighborhood, and you are alone. You quickly, but safely, stop your vehicle in front of the victim's house. When you get nearer to the victim, you notice that her skin appears bluish, and she is motionless.

Yes   No   10. Do you have to stop to help her?

____   11. If you stop and help, which type of consent would apply in this case?
  A. expressed   B. implied

Yes   No   12. If she does not respond to your tapping on her shoulders and shouting "Are you O.K.?" you can leave her and assume that someone else who is more competent or is a family member will arrive shortly to help her.

Yes   No   13. You decide to help. You straighten one of her legs, which causes a bone to protrude through the skin. Would this increase the likelihood of being sued?

Yes   No   14. For the situation in number 13, the Good Samaritan law protects you from being sued.

Yes   No   15. Rather than check the victim's breathing and pulse, you proceed to care for the broken leg. By doing so, have you failed to provide appropriate first aid?

Yes   No   16. If the woman were your mother under your custodial care, you must give first aid to her.

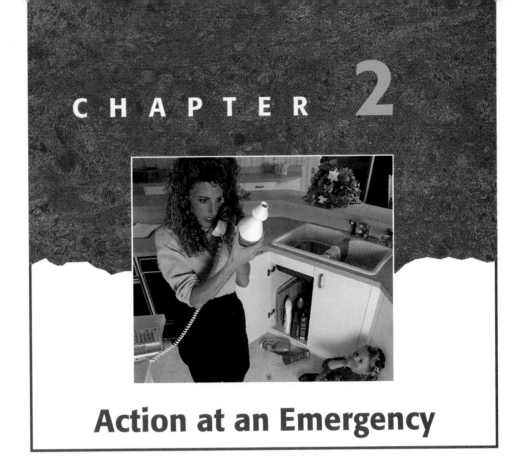

CHAPTER 2

Action at an Emergency

Bystander Intervention

The bystander is a vital link between the emergency medical service (EMS) and the victim. Typically it is a bystander who recognizes a situation as an emergency and decides to intervene to help the victim. A bystander must perform the following actions quickly and reliably.

Recognize the Emergency

To help in an emergency, the bystander first has to notice that something is wrong.

Decide to Help

Everyone will at some time have to make a decision whether to help another person. Making a quick decision to get involved at the time of an emergency is unlikely to occur unless the bystander has considered, in advance, the possibility of helping. Thus, **the most important time to make the decision to help is** *before* **you ever encounter an emergency.**

Deciding to help is an attitude about people, about emergencies, and about one's ability to deal with emergencies. It is an attitude that takes time to develop and is affected by a number of factors.

Contact the EMS, If Needed

Laypersons frequently make inappropriate decisions concerning the EMS. They delay contacting the EMS until they are absolutely sure that an emergency exists, or they elect to bypass the EMS and transport the victim to medical care in a private vehicle. Such actions can present significant dangers to victims.

Assess the Victim

The bystander must decide if life-threatening conditions exist and what kind of help a victim needs immediately.

Provide First Aid

Often the most critical life-support measures are effective only if started immediately by the nearest available person. That person usually will be a layperson—a bystander.

Post-Care Reactions

After giving first aid for severe injuries, rescuers often feel an emotional "letdown," which is frequently overlooked. Discussing your feelings, fears, and reactions within 24 to 72 hours of helping at a traumatic injury scene helps prevent later emotional problems. Such discussion may be with a trusted friend, a mental health professional, or a member of the clergy. Bringing out your feelings quickly helps to relieve personal anxieties and stress.

Scene Survey

If you are at the scene of an emergency situation, do a 10-second survey that includes looking for three things: (1) hazards that could be dangerous to you, the victim(s), or bystanders; (2) the mechanism or cause of the injury or injuries; and (3) the number of victims.

As you approach an emergency scene, scan the area for immediate dangers to yourself or to the victim. You cannot help another if you also become a victim. Always ask yourself: Is the scene safe to enter? (For details about hazards at an emergency scene, refer to Chapter 18.)

The second thing to do in the first 10 seconds is to determine the cause of the injury. Be sure to tell the EMS personnel about that, so the physician may initially be able to fully recognize the extent of the injuries.

Determine how many people are injured. There may be more than one victim, so look around and ask about others involved.

When to Call the EMS

In the following instances, calling the EMS is definitely the right thing to do:

- severe bleeding
- drowning
- electrocution
- possible heart attack
- breathing difficulty or no breathing
- choking
- altered mental status
- poisoning
- attempted suicide
- some seizure cases (most do not require EMS assistance)
- critical burns
- paralysis
- spine injury
- imminent childbirth

When a serious situation occurs, call the EMS (911 in most communities) *first*. Do *not* call your doctor, the hospital, a friend, relatives, or neighbors for help before you call the EMS. Calling anyone else first only wastes time.

If the situation is not an emergency, call your doctor. However, if you are in *any* doubt as to whether the situation is an emergency, call the EMS.

How to Call the EMS

To receive emergency assistance of every kind in most communities, you simply phone 911. Check

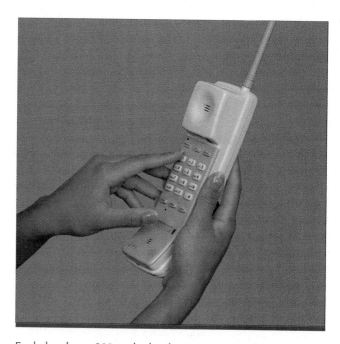

For help, phone 911 or the local emergency number.

to see if this is true in your community. Emergency telephone numbers usually are listed on the inside front cover of all telephone directories. Keep these numbers near or on every telephone. Call "O" (the operator) if you do not know the emergency number.

If you have to call the EMS, be ready to give the dispatcher the following information. Speak slowly and clearly.

1. The victim's location. Give the address, names of intersecting roads, and other landmarks, if possible. This information is the most important you can give. Also, tell the specific location of the victim (e.g., "in the basement").
2. Your phone number and name. This prevents false calls and allows a dispatch center without the enhanced 911 system to call back for additional information, if needed.
3. What happened. State the nature of the emergency (e.g., "My husband fell off a ladder and is not moving").
4. Number of persons needing help and any special conditions.
5. Victim's condition (e.g., "My husband's head is bleeding") and any first aid you have tried (such as pressing on the site of the bleeding).

Do *not* hang up the phone unless the dispatcher instructs you to do so. Enhanced 911 systems can track a call, but some communities lack this technology or are still using a seven-digit emergency number. Also, the EMS dispatcher may tell you how best to care for the victim. If you send someone else to call, have the person report back to you so you can be sure the call was made.

Disease Precautions

First aiders must be aware of the risks associated with emergency medical care. One such risk comes from infectious diseases, which can range in severity from mild to life threatening. First aiders should know how to reduce the risk of contamination to themselves and to others. This section stresses the importance of precautionary measures that help to protect against infection from disease agents such as viruses and bacteria.

Bloodborne Disease

Some diseases are caused by microorganisms that are "borne" (carried) in a person's bloodstream.

Contact with blood infected with such microorganisms may cause infection. Of the many bloodborne pathogens, three pose significant health threats to first aiders: hepatitis B virus (HBV), hepatitis C virus, and human immunodeficiency virus (HIV).

Hepatitis B

Hepatitis is a viral infection of the liver. Types A, B, and C are seen most often. Each is caused by a different virus.

A vaccine for hepatitis B is available and is recommended for all infants and for adults who may have contact with carriers of the disease or with blood. Medical and laboratory workers, police, intravenous drug users, people with multiple sexual partners, and those living with someone who has lifelong infection are at high risk of hepatitis B (and hepatitis C as well). Vaccination is the best defense against HBV. There is no chance of developing hepatitis B from the vaccine. Federal laws require employers to offer a series of three vaccine injections free to all employees who may be at risk of exposure.

Without vaccination shots, exposure to hepatitis B may produce symptoms within two weeks to six months following exposure. People with hepatitis B infection may be symptom free, but that does *not* mean they are not contagious. These people may infect others through exposure to their blood. Symptoms of hepatitis B resemble those of the flu and include fatigue, nausea, loss of appetite, stomach pain, and perhaps a yellowing of the skin.

Hepatitis B starts as an inflammation of the liver and usually lasts one to two months. In a few people, the infection is very serious, and in some, mild infection continues for life. The virus may stay in the liver and can lead to severe damage (cirrhosis) and liver cancer. Medical treatment that begins immediately after exposure may prevent infection from developing.

Hepatitis C

Hepatitis C is caused by a different virus from HBV, but both diseases have a great deal in common. Like hepatitis B, hepatitis C affects the liver and can lead to long-term liver disease and liver cancer. Hepatitis C varies in severity and may even cause no symptoms at the time of infection. Currently, there is no vaccine or effective treatment for hepatitis C.

HIV

A person infected with HIV can infect others, and HIV-infected persons almost always develop acquired immunodeficiency syndrome (AIDS), which interferes with the body's ability to fight off other diseases. No vaccine is available to prevent HIV infection, which eventually proves fatal. The best defense against AIDS is to avoid becoming infected.

Protection
In most cases, you can control the risk of exposure to bloodborne pathogens by wearing the proper PPE and by following some simple procedures.

Personal Protective Equipment (PPE)
This equipment blocks entry of an organism into the body. The most common type of protection is gloves. The Food and Drug Administration (FDA), the Centers for Disease Control and Prevention (CDC), and the Occupational Safety and Health Administration (OSHA) have stated that vinyl and latex gloves are equally protective. All first aid kits should have several pairs of gloves.

Protective eyewear and a standard surgical mask may be necessary at some emergencies; first aiders ordinarily will not have or need such equipment.

Mouth-to-barrier devices are recommended for rescue breathing and cardiopulmonary resuscitation (CPR). No case of disease transmission to a rescuer as a result of performing unprotected CPR on an infected victim has been documented. Nevertheless, a mouth-to-barrier device should be used whenever possible.

Universal Precautions or Body Substance Isolation?
Individuals infected with HBV or HIV may not show symptoms and may not even know they are infectious. For that reason, all human blood and body fluids should be considered infectious, and precautions should be taken to avoid contact. The *body substance isolation* (BSI) technique assumes that *all* body fluids are a possible risk. EMS personnel routinely follow BSI procedures, even if blood or body fluids are not visible.

OSHA requires any company with employees who are expected to give first aid in an emergency to follow *universal precautions,* which assume that *all* blood and *certain* body fluids pose a risk for transmission of HBV and HIV. OSHA considers an employee who assists another with a nosebleed or a cut to fall under the definition of "Good Samaritan." Such acts, however, are not considered occupational exposure unless the employee who provides the assistance is a member of a first aid team or is designated or expected to render first aid as part of his or her job. In essence, OSHA's requirement excludes unassigned employees who perform unanticipated first aid.

Whenever there is a chance you could be exposed to bloodborne pathogens, your employer must provide appropriate PPE, which might include eye protection, gloves, gowns, and masks. The PPE must be accessible, and your employer must provide training to help you choose the right PPE for your work.

While EMS personnel follow BSI procedures and OSHA requires designated worksite first aiders to follow universal precautions, what should a typical first aider do? It makes sense for first aiders to follow BSI procedures and assume that *all* blood and body fluids are infectious and follow appropriate protective measures.

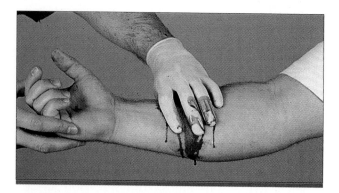

Whenever possible, use gloves as a barrier.

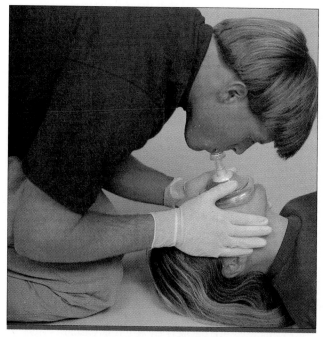

Pocket face mask, one-way valve

Coping with Emergencies

When an injury occurs, first aiders can protect themselves and others against bloodborne pathogens by following these steps:

1. Wear appropriate PPE, such as gloves.
2. If you have been trained in the correct procedures, use absorbent barriers to soak up blood or other infectious materials.
3. Clean the spill area with an appropriate disinfecting solution, such as diluted bleach.
4. Discard contaminated materials in an appropriate waste disposal container.

If you have been exposed to blood or body fluids:

1. Use soap and water to wash the parts of your body that have been contaminated.
2. If the exposure happens while at work, report the incident to your supervisor. Otherwise, contact your personal physician. Early action can prevent the development of hepatitis B and enable affected workers to track potential HIV infection.

The best protection against bloodborne disease is using the safeguards described here. By following these guidelines, first aiders can decrease their chance of contracting bloodborne illness.

Airborne Disease

Infective organisms (e.g., bacteria, viruses) that are introduced into the air by coughing or sneezing are said to be "airborne." Droplets of mucus that carry those bacteria or viruses can then be inhaled by other individuals. The rate of tuberculosis (TB) has increased recently and is receiving much attention. TB, caused by bacteria, sometimes settles in the lungs and can be fatal. In most cases, a first aider will not know that a victim has TB. Assume that any person with a cough, especially one who is in a nursing home or a shelter, may have TB. Other symptoms include fatigue, weight loss, chest pain, and coughing up blood. If a surgical mask is available, wear it or wrap a handkerchief over your nose and mouth.

Action at an Emergency

Directions: Circle Yes if you agree with the statement, and circle No if you disagree.

Yes   No   1. Everyone will at some time have to make the decision whether to help another person.

Yes   No   2. Deciding to help others should be done before encountering an emergency.

Yes   No   3. A scene survey should be done before giving first aid to an injured victim.

Yes   No   4. For a severely injured victim, first call the victim's doctor before calling for an ambulance.

Yes   No   5. Most communities use the 911 telephone number for emergencies.

Yes   No   6. First aiders should assume that blood and all body fluids are infectious.

Yes   No   7. If you have been exposed to blood while on the job, report it to your supervisor, and if off the job, your personal physician.

Yes   No   8. First aid kits should contain disposable gloves.

Scenario: You are rushing parts to one of your largest customer's broken machines. Since "time is money," the customer is losing a lot for each hour its machine is down. It's beginning to rain. Suddenly, you see a motorcyclist skidding off the country highway with the cyclist ending up in a barbwire fence alongside the highway. No other traffic is seen. You have a cellular telephone in your car.

9. Name the 5 actions that a bystander can take at an emergency.

a. _____   d. _____

b. _____   e. _____

c. _____

10. A scene survey consists of looking for what three things?

a. _____   c. _____

b. _____

11. When talking with an EMS dispatcher, what information should you expect to give?

a. _____   c. _____

b. _____   d. _____

12. How would you protect yourself against bloodborne pathogens?

a. _____   c. _____

b. _____

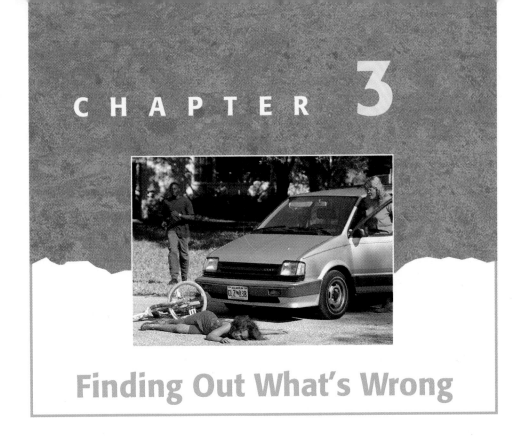

CHAPTER 3

Finding Out What's Wrong

A logical, systematic format known as **victim assessment** will help you evaluate the victim. Victim assessment is divided into three steps:

1. the primary survey to determine any life-threatening conditions
2. the physical exam to evaluate nonemergency conditions
3. the victim's history (*For a suddenly ill person you may want to complete the victim's history before conducting the physical exam.*)

After you have determined that the situation is safe (see page 6), you can perform the primary survey. Make all assessments while close to the victim.

If two or more people are injured, attend to the quiet one first. A quiet victim may not have an open airway or a pulse. A victim who is talking, crying, or yelling obviously has an open airway.

Most injured or ill victims do not require a complete victim assessment. The circumstances of the same type of injury usually will determine if a complete assessment is necessary. For example, a victim who cuts a finger while peeling a potato won't require a complete assessment, but a victim with a cut finger from a bicycle collision will because other injuries may be present.

The Primary Survey

The goal of the primary survey is to quickly assess the heart, lungs, brain, and spinal cord which are essential to life. Any life-threatening condition, such as an obstructed airway or massive bleeding, found during the primary survey must be corrected before you continue the victim assessment. Since most injured victims won't have life-threatening conditions, most primary surveys will be completed quickly.

First, form a general impression of the victim based on an immediate assessment of the scene and the victim's chief complaint. Look at the surroundings

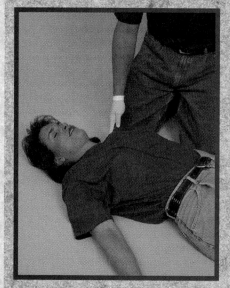

1.

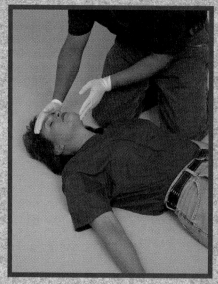

2.

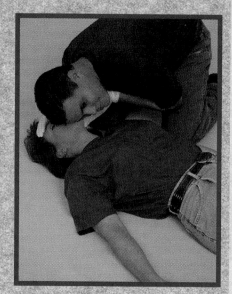

3.

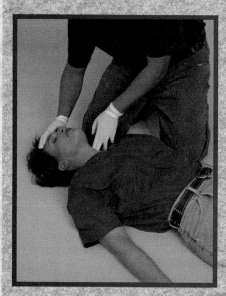

4a.

1. Responsive?
2. A = Airway open?
3. B = Breathing?
4. C = Circulation
    a. Carotid pulse?
    b. Hemorrhage/severe bleeding?
    c. Condition of skin? (not shown)
      • color
      • temperature
      • moisture
5. D = Disability
    • spinal cord response
    • mental status

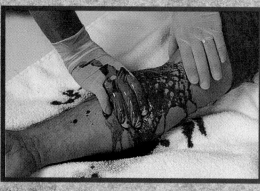

4b.

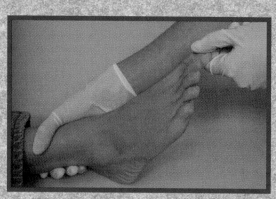

5.

PRIMARY SURVEY

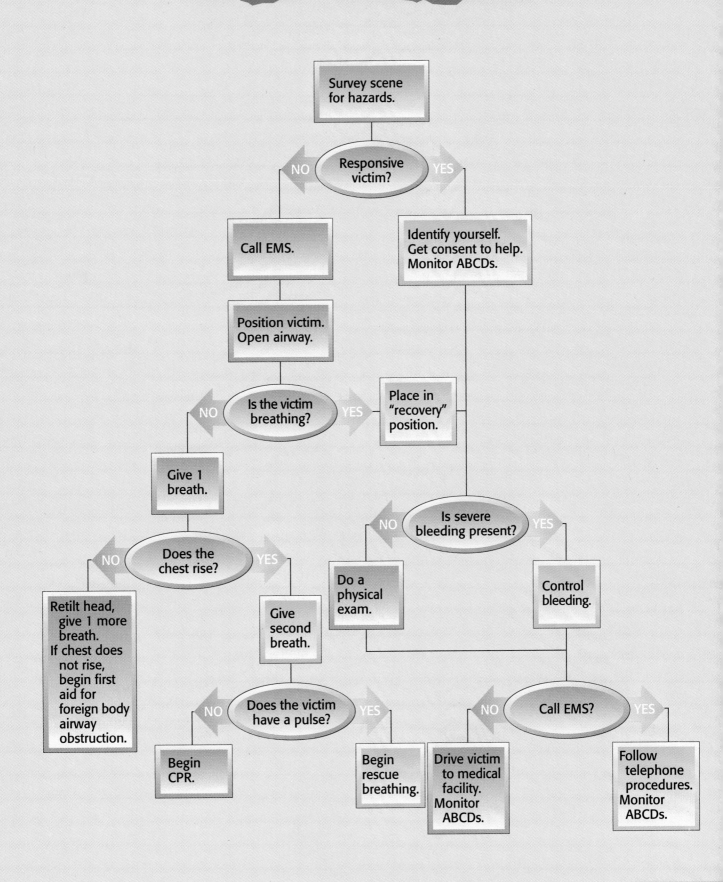

Survey scene for hazards.

Responsive victim?

NO → Call EMS.

Position victim. Open airway.

Is the victim breathing?

NO → Give 1 breath.

Does the chest rise?

NO → Retilt head, give 1 more breath. If chest does not rise, begin first aid for foreign body airway obstruction.

YES → Give second breath.

Does the victim have a pulse?

NO → Begin CPR.

YES → Begin rescue breathing.

YES → Place in "recovery" position.

YES → Identify yourself. Get consent to help. Monitor ABCDs.

Is severe bleeding present?

NO → Do a physical exam.

YES → Control bleeding.

Call EMS?

NO → Drive victim to medical facility. Monitor ABCDs.

YES → Follow telephone procedures. Monitor ABCDs.

and the mechanisms of injury (MOI). Then assess the victim's responsiveness or mental status. Begin by asking if he or she is okay. State your name, tell the victim you are a first aider, and explain that you are there to help. Then gain consent by asking if you can help. If you suspect a spine injury, stabilize the spine against moving.

A: Open the Airway

If the victim is talking or responsive, the airway is open. For an unresponsive victim, open the airway with the head-tilt/chin-lift method unless you suspect a spine injury (see page 25).

B: Assess Breathing

Responsive victims are breathing. Note any breathing difficulties or unusual breathing sounds such as wheezing, crowing, gurgling, or snoring. If the victim is unresponsive, keep the airway open and look for the chest to rise and fall, listen for breathing, and feel for air coming out of the victim's nose and mouth. If there is no breathing, give two breaths. (Refer to page 25 for details.) If an unresponsive victim is breathing, place the victim on his or her left side (recovery position, see page 22).

C: Assess Circulation

First, check an unresponsive victim's pulse by feeling at the side of the neck (carotid artery) or, for an infant, at the upper arm (brachial artery). If a pulse

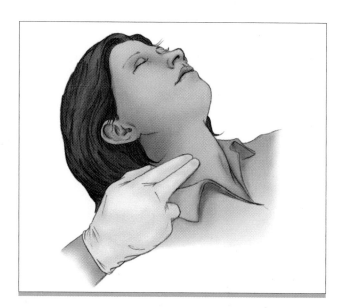

Palpating (feeling) the carotid pulse

is absent, cardiopulmonary resuscitation (CPR) is required. If a pulse is present, but there is no breathing, give rescue breathing. Refer to page 26 for details.

Second, check for major bleeding by looking over the victim's entire body for blood (blood-soaked clothing or blood pooling on the floor or the ground). Bleeding requires the application of direct pressure or a pressure bandage. Avoid contact with the victim's blood, if possible, by using latex gloves or extra layers of cloth or dressings. Control any bleeding as described on pages 39–41.

Finally, check the victim's skin condition (color, temperature, and moisture). Skin color, especially in light-skinned people, reflects the circulation under the skin as well as oxygen status. In darkly pigmented people, changes may not be readily apparent but can be assessed by the appearance of the nail beds, the inside of the mouth, and the inner eyelids. When the skin's blood vessels constrict or the pulse slows, the skin becomes cool and pale or cyanotic (blue-gray color). When the skin's blood vessels dilate or blood flow increases, the skin becomes warm.

You can get a rough idea of temperature by putting the back of your hand or wrist on the victim's forehead and your other hand on your own forehead or that of another healthy person. If the victim has a fever, you should feel the difference. Abnormal skin temperature will feel hot, cool, cold, or clammy (cool and moist).

Notice if the skin seems dry (normal) or moist or wet (abnormal).

D: Assess Disability

Check for a spine injury, especially if the victim has been injured in a fall, a motor vehicle crash, or other incident that could produce a spine injury. Assume that a victim with a head injury has a spine injury until it is proved otherwise. To assess a victim for a spine injury: (1) check sensation by squeezing the victim's fingers and toes; (2) check movement by having the victim wiggle his or her fingers and toes; and (3) have the victim perform a hand squeeze and a foot push. See page 83 for details.

If you suspect a spine injury, do not move the victim's head or neck. See page 85 for the best way to stabilize a neck at the accident scene.

Next, check the victim's level of responsiveness. Avoid using confusing terms such as "semiconscious" and "in and out" to describe the victim's responsiveness. Instead, use one of four levels on the AVPU scale.

A victim's level of responsiveness or mental status can be described according to the following AVPU scale. The V, P, and U levels can help determine damage from decreased oxygen to the brain, drug or alcohol overdose, central nervous system (CNS) injury, or metabolic derangement from diabetes, a seizure, or a heart condition.

> **A**: **A**lert. The victim's eyes are open, and he or she can answer questions clearly. A victim who knows the date (*time*), where he or she is (*place*), and his or her own name (*person*) is said to be alert.
>
> **V**: Responsive to **V**erbal stimulus. The victim may not be oriented to time, place, and person but does respond in some meaningful way when spoken to.
>
> **P**: Responsive only to **P**ainful stimulus. The eyes do not open, and the victim does not respond to questions. The victim does respond to your pinching of the skin over the collarbone.
>
> **U**: **U**nresponsive to any stimulus. The eyes do not open, and the victim does not respond to pinching of the skin.

E: Expose the Injury

Clothing can hide an injury. How much clothing you should remove varies, depending on the victim's condition and injuries. The general rule is to remove as much clothing as necessary to determine the presence or absence of a condition or an injury. Keep in mind that most injured victims are susceptible to hypothermia. If the removal of certain items of clothing may prove embarrassing to the victim or to bystanders, explain what you intend to do and why.

The Physical Exam

After you have completed the primary survey and attended to any life-threatening conditions, next make a systematic physical exam. The physical exam will uncover injuries or illnesses that, while not posing an immediate threat to life, may do so if they remain uncorrected. Even minor injuries need treatment, but first they must be found. If there are two or more victims, complete the primary survey on each before checking either with a physical exam.

Carry out a physical exam while close to the victim. Standing over someone lying on the ground sends the signal to the victim and to others that you want to keep your clothes clean or that you do not really want to help.

By now, you will have a good idea whether the victim's condition involves an injury or a sudden illness. The physical exam of a victim with a sudden illness focuses on a particular complaint. The physical exam of an injured victim may focus on a specific part of the body. Make sure you tell the victim what you are doing and why.

··

⚠ CAUTION: DO NOT

- aggravate injuries or contaminate wounds.
- move a victim with a possible spine injury.

··

Systematically start a "looking and feeling" exam at the victim's head and proceed down the body to the feet. With children, start at their feet, since it is less frightening to them. The mnemonic LAF can remind you how to examine an area:

> **L**: **L**ook at the area for deformity, open wounds, and swelling.
>
> **A**: **A**nd
>
> **F**: **F**eel for deformity, tenderness, and swelling.

Use the mnemonic DOTS to remember the signs of injury:

> **D**: **D**eformity
>
> **O**: **O**pen wounds
>
> **T**: **T**enderness
>
> **S**: **S**welling

Use the LAF method to briefly inspect (look at) and palpate (feel) the following body areas in a logical manner: head, neck, chest, abdomen, pelvis, and all four extremities. Use DOTS to locate any injuries.

The following checklist indicates some of the things you should look and feel for:

■ Head	Deformity?
	Open wounds?
	Tenderness?
	Swelling?
	Cerebrospinal fluid (CSF, a clear fluid) from ear or nose?
■ Eyes	Use the mnemonic PEARL (**P**upils **E**qual **A**nd **R**eact to **L**ight). Use a flashlight or

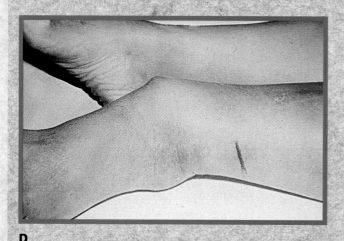

D

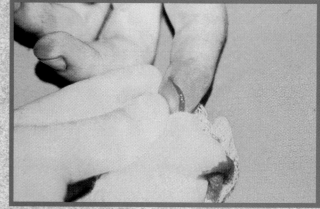

O

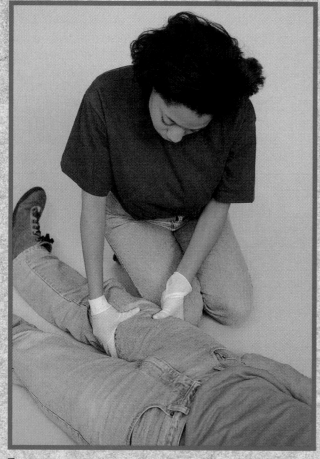

T

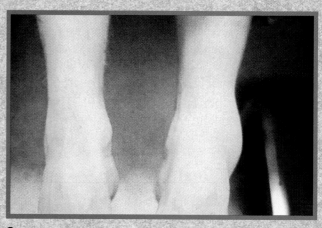

S

Examine an area by looking and feeling (LAF) for deformity, open wounds, tenderness, and swelling (DOTS).

D = Deformity
O = Open wounds
T = Tenderness
S = Swelling

SKILL SCAN: Physical Exam—Injury

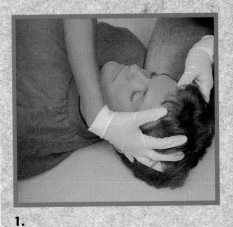

1.

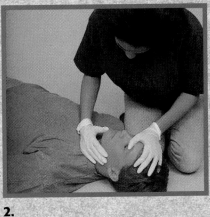

2.

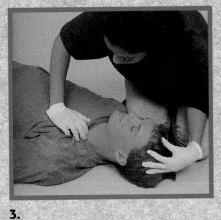

3.

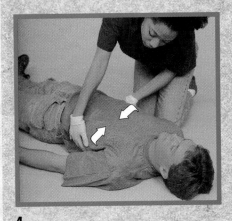

4.

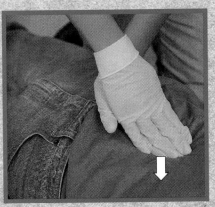

5.

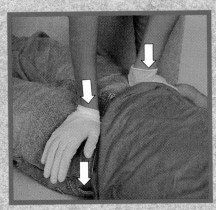

6a.

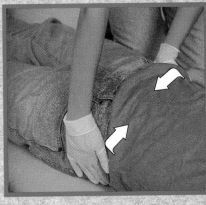

6b.

Briefly inspect by looking and feeling:

1. Head: DOTS; cerebrospinal fluid
2. Eyes: PEARL—Pupils are Equal And React to Light
3. Neck: DOTS
4. Chest: DOTS; squeeze chest
5. Abdomen: DOTS; gently press abdomen
6. Pelvis: a. Gently press downward
   b. Gently squeeze inward
7. Extremities: DOTS arms and legs; check CSM—Circulation, Sensation, Movement

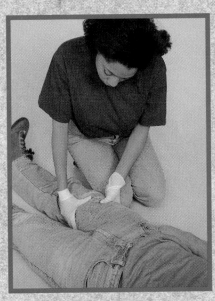

7.

cover and then uncover the victim's eyes with your hand to determine if the pupils are reactive (i.e., they constrict in response to light). Unequal pupils occur normally in 2 to 4 percent of the population but should be of equal size when the brain is not injured.

- Neck — Deformity?

  Open wounds?

  Tenderness?

  Swelling?

- Chest — Deformity?

  Open wounds?

  Tenderness? (Squeeze or compress the sides for rib pain.)

  Swelling?

- Abdomen — Deformity?

  Open wounds?

  Tenderness? (Gently press the four abdominal quadrants for firmness and softness.)

  Swelling?

- Pelvis — Deformity?

  Open wounds?

  Tenderness? (Gently press downward and squeeze inward.)

  Swelling?

- Extremities — Deformity?

  Open wounds?

  Tenderness?

  Swelling?

  Circulation, Sensation, and Movement (CSM) (See pages 94–96.)

The Victim's History

The interview usually involves the victim, but it may include the family and bystanders if the victim is unresponsive or a young child.

Ask the victim about his or her condition. Those with chronic health problems can often tell you what is best for them.

Question the victim or the victim's family, if time permits, to learn the victim's relevant medical history. The information gained may indicate what is wrong or what needs to be passed along to medical personnel. Use the mnemonic SAMPLE to help you collect the victim's history.

Note: For suddenly ill victims, you may want to collect the SAMPLE history before you conduct the physical exam.

S: **S**igns and symptoms. A sign is any condition or injury *displayed* by the victim and identifiable by the first aider (e.g., bleeding, skin temperature). A symptom is any condition *described* by the victim (e.g., headache, stomachache). As you locate signs and symptoms of illness or injury, there may be specific questions that you as a first aider should ask (described in later chapters on illness and injury).

A: **A**llergies. "Are you allergic to anything?" The answer may give a clue as to the problem.

M: **M**edications. "Do you take any prescription or over-the-counter medicine?" The answer may give a clue as to the problem and help prevent the administration of contraindicated medication.

P: **P**ertinent past illnesses. "Are you seeing a doctor for anything?" (relating to the present problem)

L: **L**ast oral intake. "When was the last time you had anything to eat or drink? How much? Was it solid or liquid?" The answers are important in case surgery is necessary or food poisoning is suspected.

E: **E**vents leading to the injury or illness. "What were you doing when this happened?"

Medical Identification Tags

Look for medical identification tags, which may be beneficial in identifying allergies, medications, or medical history. A medical-alert tag, worn as a necklace or as a bracelet, contains the wearer's medical problem(s) and a 24-hour telephone number that offers, in case of an emergency, access to the

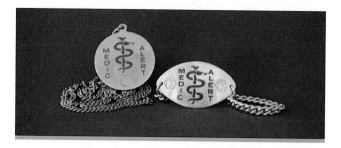

Medical-alert tag

victim's medical history plus names of doctors and close relatives. Necklaces and bracelets are durable, instantly recognizable, and less likely than cards to be separated from the victim in an emergency.

Putting It All Together

The victim assessment will be influenced by whether the victim is suffering from a sudden illness or from an injury, whether the victim is responsive or unresponsive, and whether life-threatening conditions are present. Be sure to conduct a primary survey and correct any life-threatening problem *before* going on to the physical exam and the victim's history.

Medical personnel at all levels follow a systematic method of assessing an injured person. The assessment methods may vary, but all share a similar format. The method presented here can help you during those hectic, panicky, emergency situations when you may be wondering what to do first.

While you are waiting for an ambulance, continue to check the victim. Ongoing assessment allows you to calm and reassure the victim and at the same time to reassess the ABCDs. Repeat the primary assessment every 15 minutes for a responsive victim and every 5 minutes for an unresponsive victim. Use the AVPU scale to check the victim's mental status. Check any first aid that has been given, including bandages and splints.

When the ambulance arrives, report to the emergency medical personnel the following information:

1. victim's chief complaint
2. responsiveness (AVPU scale)
3. ABCD (airway, breathing, circulation, disability) status
4. physical exam findings
5. SAMPLE history
6. any first aid that has been provided

Victim-Assessment Checklist

1. **Scene Survey**
   Hazards?
   Number of victims?
   Mechanism (cause) of injury?
2. **Primary Survey**
   A = Airway open?
   B = Breathing?
   C = Circulation
   - carotid pulse?
   - hemorrhage?
   - skin condition (temperature, moisture, color)
   D = Disability?
   - spine injury?
   - mental status on AVPU scale?
3. **Physical Exam**
   Head: DOTS, CSF
   Eyes: PEARL
   Neck: DOTS
   Chest: DOTS (squeeze)
   Abdomen: DOTS (push)
   Pelvis: DOTS (squeeze and push)
   Extremities: DOTS, CSM
4. **Victim's History** (for sudden illness, may be completed before physical exam)
   SAMPLE
   Medical-alert tag?

Finding Out What's Wrong

Directions: Circle Yes if you agree with the statement, and circle No if you disagree.

Yes No 1. A primary survey's purpose is to find life-threatening conditions.

Yes No 2. Crying or screaming victims should be treated before quiet ones.

Yes No 3. Most injured victims require a complete victim assessment.

Yes No 4. In a physical exam, you usually begin at the head and work down the body.

Yes No 5. The mnemonic AVPU is useful for determining the victim's level of responsiveness.

Yes No 6. The mnemonic DOTS helps in remembering what to collect about the victim's history that may be useful.

Yes No 7. For all injured and suddenly ill persons, look for medical-alert identification.

Yes No 8. The mnemonic SAMPLE can remind you how to examine an area for signs of an injury.

Scenario: During a mid-morning break, a co-worker screams that somebody has collapsed in the hallway. As a company designated first aider, you push your way through a crowd of people gathered around the victim. You recognize Clyde, one of the older employees who is about to retire from the company, lying on the floor motionless. You notice that he wears a medical-alert identification bracelet.

_____ 9. After confirming that the scene is safe, you next check Clyde for:
   A. breathing   B. pulse   C. broken bones   D. responsiveness

_____10. If he were unresponsive, you:
   A. open his airway and check for breathing   C. look and feel for broken bones
   B. feel for a neck pulse   D. look at his medical-alert ID tag

_____11. If Clyde were responsive and breathing, what would you next check?
   A. physical exam   B. disability (spine injury)   C. victim's history

_____12. For injured victims, which usually comes first?
   A. physical exam   B. victim's history

_____13. The physical exam on an adult should be started at the victim's:
   A. head   B. chest   C. feet

_____14. Which of these would the medical-alert identification bracelet help identify?
   A. allergies   B. medications   C. medical history   D. all of these

_____15. When checking Clyde's eyes, you should look for:
   A. color of the iris   C. equal or unequal size of the pupils
   B. reaction of pupils to light   D. both B and C

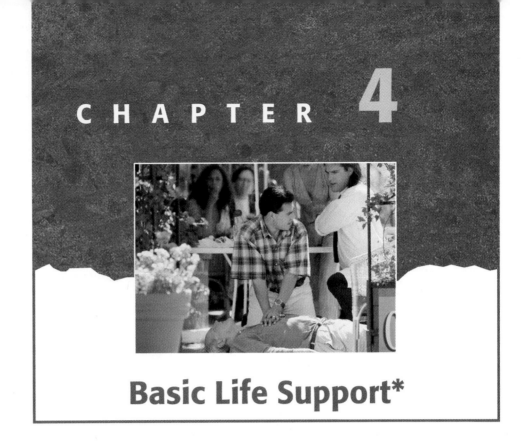

CHAPTER 4

Basic Life Support*

Heart attacks causing heart stoppage (cardiac arrest) are the most prominent cause of death in North America. In addition, drownings, suffocations, electrocutions, and drug intoxication cause cardiac arrest. Many deaths could be prevented if the victims got prompt help—if someone trained in CPR provided proper life-saving measures until trained EMS professionals could take over.

Adult and Child Basic Life Support

For the nonbreathing victim, rescue breathing must be started immediately. This is one of the most important procedures that you as a first aider will be called on to do. For best results, you must understand the process so well that you can proceed automatically.

Rescue Breathing

Place a breathing unconscious victim in the recovery position (see page 22). If a victim is not breathing, perform rescue breathing by using one of the following methods: mouth-to-mouth, mouth-to-nose, mouth-to-stoma, or mouth-to-barrier device.

Mouth-to-Mouth Method
The mouth-to-mouth method of rescue breathing is the simplest, quickest, and most effective method for an emergency situation.

Do not remove a victim's dentures unless they interfere with rescue breathing. Even loose dentures give form and shape to the victim's mouth.

*Based on the American Heart Association, Guidelines for Cardiopulmonary Resuscitation and Emergency Cardiac Care, *JAMA,* 268: 2172 (1992).

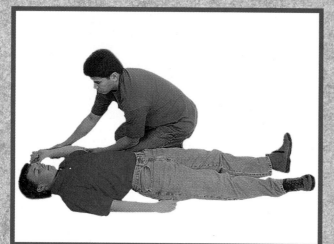

1.

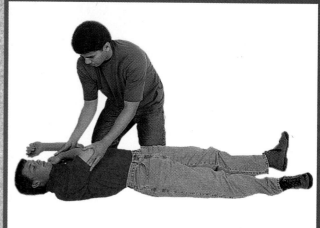

2.

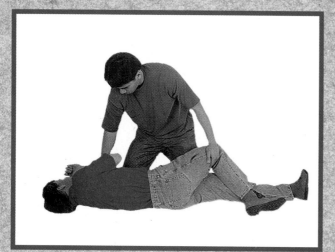

3.

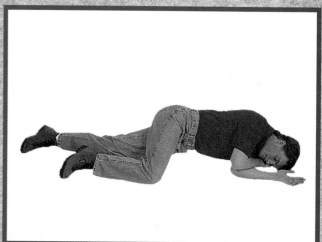

4.

1. Bend arm. Keep legs straight.
2. Place back of victim's hand against cheek and hold there.
3. Hold victim's hand against cheek to support head. Pull bent leg and roll victim toward you.
4. Hand supports head. Bent knee prevents rolling. Bent arm gives stability. Front view of recovery position.

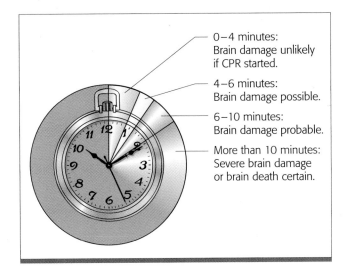

0–4 minutes:
Brain damage unlikely
if CPR started.

4–6 minutes:
Brain damage possible.

6–10 minutes:
Brain damage probable.

More than 10 minutes:
Severe brain damage
or brain death certain.

Start resuscitation efforts at once. Brain damage occurs without oxygen.

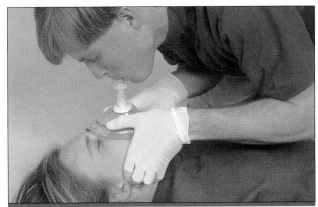

Mouth-to-barrier device

Mouth-to-Nose Method

Although mouth-to-mouth breathing is successful in the majority of cases, certain complications necessitate mouth-to-nose rescue breathing: the victim's mouth cannot be opened, teeth clenched together, a good seal cannot be made around the victim's mouth, the victim's mouth is severely injured, or the victim's mouth is too large or has no teeth.

The mouth-to-nose technique is performed like mouth-to-mouth breathing, except that you force your exhaled breath through the victim's nose while holding his or her mouth closed with one hand pushing up on the chin. The victim's mouth then must be held open so any nasal obstruction does not impede exhalation of air from the victim's lungs.

Mouth-to-Stoma Method

Cancer and other diseases of the vocal cords often make surgical removal of the larynx necessary. Breathing is through a small permanent opening called a *stoma,* which is surgically made in the lower part of the neck and joined to the trachea.

In mouth-to-stoma rescue breathing, the victim's mouth and nose must be closed during the delivery of breaths because the air can flow upward into the upper airway through the larynx as well as downward into the lungs. You can close the victim's mouth and nose with one hand. Determine breathing by looking at, listening to, and feeling the stoma. Keep the victim's head and neck level.

Mouth-to-Barrier Device

A mouth-to-barrier device is an apparatus that is placed over a victim's face as a safety precaution for the rescuer during rescue breathing. There are two types of mouth-to-barrier devices:

- *Face masks.* Face masks cover the victim's mouth and nose. Most have a one-way valve so exhaled air from the victim does not enter the rescuer's mouth. According to the American Heart Association, face masks are more effective than face shields.

- *Face shields.* These clear plastic devices have a mouthpiece through which the rescuer breathes. Some models have a short airway that is inserted into the victim's mouth over the tongue. They are smaller and less expensive than face masks, but air can leak around the shield. Also, they cover only the victim's mouth, so the nose must be pinched. The American Heart Association recommends replacing face shields with face masks as soon as possible.

Use of a barrier device requires the victim's neck to be hyperextended and the chin lifted. After the mask is in place, the rescuer breathes through the device. The technique is performed like mouth-to-mouth breathing.

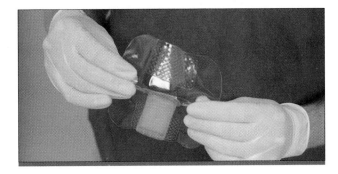

Face shield

If you see a motionless person . . .

1

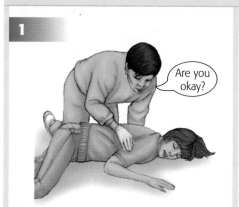

Check responsiveness

- If spine injury is suspected, move victim only if absolutely necessary.
- Tap victim's shoulder.
- Shout near victim's ear, "Are you okay?"

2

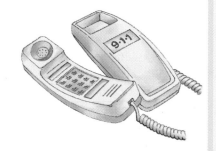

Activate the EMS for help

- Ask a bystander to call the local emergency telephone number, usually 911.
- If you are alone, shout for help. If no one comes quickly, call the local emergency telephone number. If someone does come quickly, ask him or her to call.

For a child (1–8 years)

- If you are alone, call the EMS after 1 minute of resuscitation unless a nearby bystander can be sent.

3

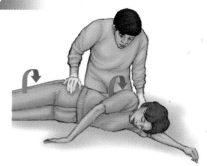

Roll person onto back

- Gently roll victim's head, body, and legs over at the same time. Do this without further injuring the victim.

4

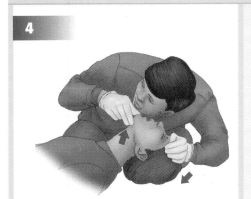

Open airway (use head-tilt/chin-lift method)
- Place your hand that is nearest victim's head on victim's forehead and apply backward pressure to tilt head back.
- Place fingers of your other hand under bony part of jaw near chin and lift. Avoid pressing on soft tissues under jaw.
- Tilt head backward without closing victim's mouth.
- Do *not* use your thumb to lift the chin.

If you suspect a spine injury

Do *not* move victim's head or neck. First try lifting chin without tilting head back. If breaths do not go in, slowly and gently bend the head back until breaths go in.

5

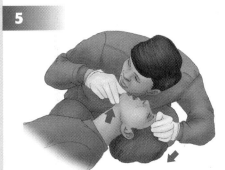

Check for breathing (take 3–5 seconds)
- Place your ear over victim's mouth and nose while keeping airway open.
- *Look* at victim's chest to check for rise and fall; *listen* and *feel* for breathing.

6

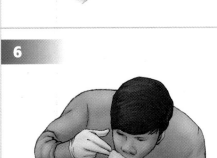

Give 2 slow breaths
- Keep head tilted back with head-tilt/chin-lift to keep airway open.
- Pinch nose shut.
- Take a deep breath and seal your lips tightly around victim's mouth.
- Give 2 slow breaths, each lasting 1½ to 2 seconds (you should take a breath after each breath given to victim).
- Watch chest rise to see if your breaths go in.
- Allow for chest deflation after each breath.

If first breath did not go in

Retilt the head and try another breath. If second breath is unsuccessful, suspect choking, also known as foreign body airway obstruction (use *Unconscious Adult and Child Foreign Body Airway Obstruction* procedures, described later in this chapter).

7

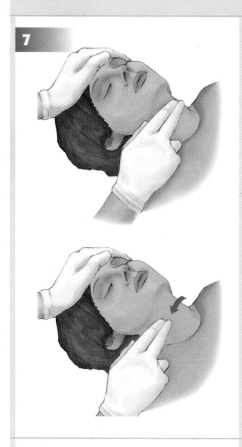

Check for pulse (take 5–10 seconds)

- Maintain head tilt with your hand nearest the victim's head on forehead.
- Locate Adam's apple with 2 or 3 fingers of hand nearer victim's feet.
- Slide your fingers down into groove of neck on side closest to you (do not use your thumb because you may feel your own pulse).
- Feel for carotid pulse (take 5–10 seconds). Carotid artery is used because it lies close to the heart and is accessible.

8

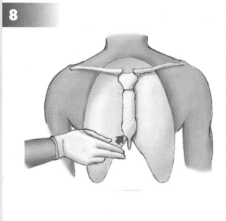

Perform rescue procedures based on what you found:

If there is a pulse but no breathing

Give one rescue breath every 5 to 6 seconds. Use the same techniques for rescue breathing given in Step 6 but give only one. Every minute (10 to 12 breaths) stop and check the pulse to make sure there is a pulse. For a child: give 1 breath every 3 seconds lasting 1 to 1½ seconds. Check the pulse every 20 breaths. Continue until:

- Victim starts breathing on his or her own.

OR

- Trained help, such as emergency medical technicians (EMTs), arrives and relieves you.

OR

- You are completely exhausted.

If there is no pulse, give CPR

- Find hand position:

    1. Slide the fingers of your hand nearest the victim's feet up rib cage edge nearer to you to notch at the end of sternum.

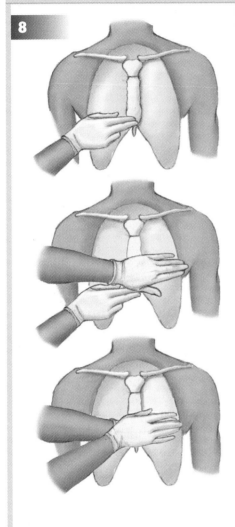

8

2. Place your middle finger on or in the notch and the index finger next to it.

3. Put heel of other hand (one closer to victim's head) on sternum next to index finger.

4. Remove hand from notch and put it on top of hand on chest.

5. Interlace, hold, or extend fingers up.

- Do 15 compressions.

  1. Place your shoulders directly over your hands on the chest.

  2. Keep arms straight and elbows locked.

  3. Push sternum straight down 1½ to 2 inches.

  4. Do 15 compressions at a rate of 80 per minute. Count as you push down: "One and, two and, three and, four and, five and, six and, seven and, . . . , fifteen and."

  5. Push smoothly; do not jerk or jab; do not stop at the top or at the bottom of the compression action.

  6. When pushing, bend from your hips, not knees.

  7. Keep fingers pointing across victim's chest, away from you.

- Give 2 slow breaths.

- Complete 3 more cycles of 15 compressions and 2 breaths (takes about 1 minute), then check the pulse. *If there is no pulse*, restart CPR with chest compressions. Recheck the pulse every few minutes. *If there is a pulse*, give rescue breathing.

- Continue CPR until:

  Victim revives.

  OR

  Trained help, such as emergency medical technicians (EMTs), arrives and relieves you.

  OR

  You are completely exhausted.

For a child

- Compress sternum with 1 hand with other hand on child's forehead.

- Compression rate to 100 times per minute. Count as you push down, "one, two, three, four, five."

- Compress 1 to 1½ inches.

- Give 1 breath after every 5 chest compressions.

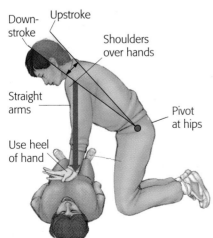

Down-stroke Upstroke

Shoulders over hands

Straight arms

Pivot at hips

Use heel of hand

Airway Obstruction (Choking) —Adult and Child

Recognizing Choking

A foreign body lodged in the airway may cause partial or complete airway obstruction. When a foreign body partially blocks the airway, either good or poor air exchange may result. When good air exchange is present, the victim is able to make forceful coughing efforts in an attempt to relieve the obstruction. The victim should be permitted and encouraged to cough. Sometimes, a good air exchange may progress to a poor air exchange.

A choking victim who has poor air exchange has weak and ineffective coughs, and breathing becomes more difficult. The skin, the fingernail beds, and the inside of the mouth may appear bluish-gray in color. Each attempt to inhale is usually accompanied by a high-pitched noise. A partial airway obstruction with poor air exchange should be treated as if it were a complete airway blockage.

Complete airway obstruction in a conscious victim commonly occurs when the victim has been eating. The victim is unable to speak, breathe, or cough. When asked, "Can you speak?" the victim is unable to respond verbally. Choking victims with complete foreign body obstruction of the airway may instinctively reach up and clutch their necks to communicate that they are choking. This motion is known as the distress signal for choking. The victim becomes panicked and desperate and may appear pale in color. Because a complete obstruction prevents air from entering the lungs, oxygen deprivation occurs within a few minutes.

Infant Basic Life Support

Basic life support techniques for an infant differ from those for an adult or child. Initially occurring cardiac arrest in infants is rare. Usually, infants have a respiratory arrest with cardiac arrest developing later because the heart muscle did not receive sufficient oxygen.

Airway Obstruction—Infant

People, especially children and infants, inhale all kinds of objects. Foods such as hot dogs, candy, peanuts, and grapes are major offenders because of their shape and consistencies. Non-food choking deaths are caused by balloons, balls and marbles, toys, and coins.

As discussed before, the airway may be partially or completely blocked. With a partial airway obstruction, an infant is able to make persistent coughing efforts that should not be hampered. If good air exchange becomes a poor exchange or poor air exchange occurs initially, the victim should be managed as having a complete airway obstruction. Poor air exchanges are indicated by ineffective coughing, high-pitched noises, breathing difficulty, and blueness of the lips and fingernail beds.

If person is conscious and cannot speak, breathe, or cough . . .

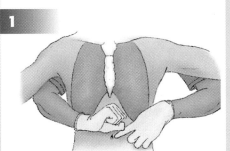

1

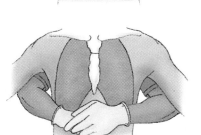

Give up to 5 abdominal thrusts (Heimlich maneuver)

- Stand behind the victim.
- Wrap your arms around victim's waist. (Do not allow your forearms to touch the ribs.)
- Make a fist with 1 hand and place the thumb side just above the victim's navel and well below the tip of the sternum.
- Grasp fist with your other hand.
- Press fist into victim's abdomen with 5 quick upward thrusts.
- Each thrust should be a separate and distinct effort to dislodge the object.

After every 5 abdominal thrusts, check the victim and your technique.

Note: If the victim is obese or in an advanced stage of pregnancy, consider using chest thrusts.

2

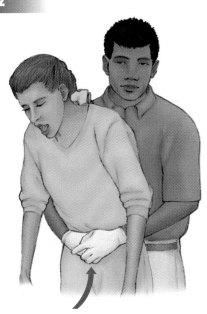

Repeat cycles of up to 5 abdominal thrusts until

- Victim coughs up object.

OR

- Victim starts to breathe or coughs forcefully.

OR

- Victim becomes unconscious (activate EMS and start methods for an unconscious victim with a finger sweep first).

OR

- You are relieved by EMS or other trained person. Reassess victim and your technique after every 5 thrusts.

If person is unconscious and breaths have not gone in . . .

1

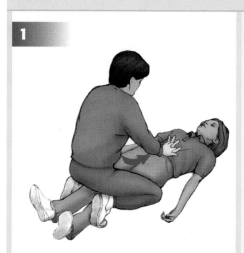

Give up to 5 abdominal thrusts (Heimlich maneuver)

- Straddle victim's thighs.
- Put heel of one hand against middle of victim's abdomen slightly above navel and well below sternum's notch (fingers of hand should point toward victim's head).
- Put other hand directly on top of first hand.
- Press inward and upward using both hands with up to 5 quick abdominal thrusts.
- Each thrust should be a separate and distinct effort to relieve the airway obstruction. Keep heel of hand in contact with abdomen between abdominal thrusts.

Note: If the victim is obese or in an advanced stage of pregnancy, consider using chest thrusts.

2

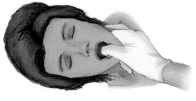

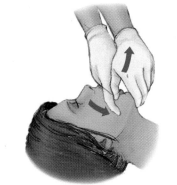

Perform finger sweep

- Use only on an unconscious victim. On a conscious victim, it may cause gagging or vomiting.
- Use your thumb and fingers to grasp victim's jaw and tongue and lift upward to pull tongue away from back of throat and away from foreign object.
- If you are unable to open mouth to perform the tongue-jaw lift, use the crossed-finger method by crossing the index finger and thumb and pushing the teeth apart.
- With index finger of your other hand, slide finger down along the inside of one cheek deeply into mouth and use a hooking action across to other cheek to dislodge foreign object.
- If foreign body comes within reach, grab and remove it. Do not force object deeper

For a child: Use finger sweep only if foreign object is seen.

3

If Steps 1 and 2 are unsuccessful
Cycle through the following steps in rapid sequence until the object is expelled or EMS arrives:

- Give 1 rescue breath.
- Do up to 5 abdominal thrusts.
- Do a finger sweep

If you see a motionless infant . . .

1

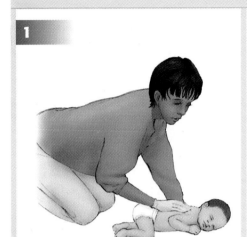

Check responsiveness
- If spine injury is suspected, move only if absolutely necessary.
- Tap infant's shoulder.

2

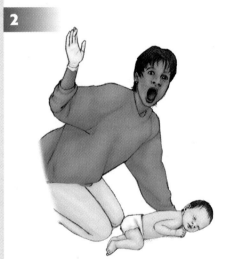

Send bystander, if available, to activate EMS. If you are alone, give rescue breathing or CPR for 1 minute before activating EMS.

3

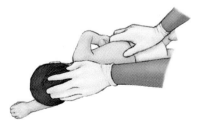

Roll infant onto back
Gently roll infant's head, body, and legs over at the same time (avoid twisting).

4

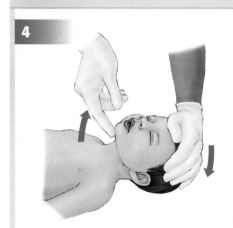

Open airway (use head-tilt/chin-lift method)
- Place your hand nearest infant's head on infant's forehead and apply backward pressure to tilt head back (known as the "sniffing" or neutral position).
- Place fingers of other hand under bony part of jaw near chin and lift. Avoid pressing on soft tissues under jaw.
- Tilt head backward without closing infant's mouth.
- Do not use your thumb to lift the chin.

If you suspect a spine injury

Do not move infant's head or neck. First try lifting chin without tilting head back. If breaths do not go in, slowly and gently bend the head back until breaths can go in.

5

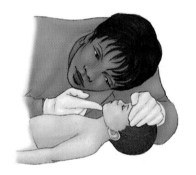

Check for breathing (take 3–5 seconds)
- Place your ear over infant's mouth and nose while keeping airway open.
- Look at infant's chest to check for rise and fall; listen and feel for breathing.

6

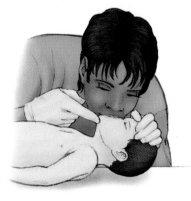

Give 2 slow breaths
- Keep head tilted back with head-tilt/chin-lift to keep airway open.
- With your mouth make a seal over infant's mouth and nose.
- Give 2 slow breaths, each lasting 1 to 1½ seconds (you should take a breath after each breath given).
- Watch chest rise to see if your breaths go in.
- Allow for chest deflation after each breath.

If first breath did not go in

Retilt the head and try another breath. If second breath is unsuccessful, suspect choking, also known as foreign body airway obstruction (refer to the *Unconscious Infant with Foreign Body Airway Obstruction(Choking)* section).

7

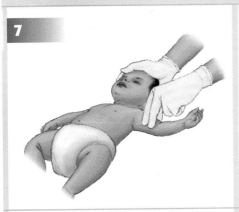

Check for pulse

- Maintain head tilt with hand nearest head on forehead.
- Feel for pulse on the inside of the upper arm between the elbow and armpit (the brachial).
- Press gently with 2 fingers on inside of arm closest to you.
- Place thumb of same hand on outside of infant's upper arm.

8

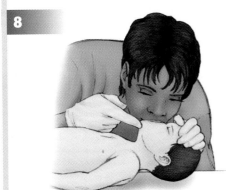

Perform rescue procedures based on your pulse check.

If there is a pulse but no breathing

Give rescue breaths every 3 seconds. Use the same techniques for rescue breathing given in Step 6 but give only one breath. If you are alone, activate the EMS after the first minute. Every minute (20 breaths), stop and check the pulse to make sure there is one. Continue until:

- Infant starts breathing on his or her own.

OR

- Trained help, such as emergency medical technicians (EMTs), arrives and relieves you.

OR

- You are completely exhausted.

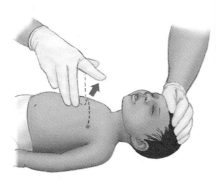

If there is no pulse, give CPR

- Locate fingers' position.
  1. Maintain a head tilt.
  2. Imagine a line connecting the nipples.
  3. Place 3 fingers on sternum with index finger touching but below imaginary nipple line.
  4. Raise your index finger and use other 2 fingers for compression. If you feel the notch at the end of the sternum, move your fingers up a little.
- Give 5 compressions.
  1. Do 5 chest compressions at rate of 100 per minute. Count as you push down, "one, two, three, four, five."
  2. Press sternum ½ to 1 inch or about ⅓ to ½ of the depth of the chest.
  3. Keep fingers pointing across the infant's chest away from you. Keep fingers in contact with infant's chest.
  4. Maintain head tilt with hand nearest head on forehead.

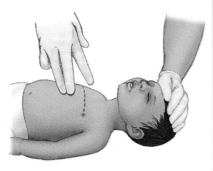

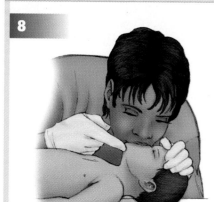

8

- Give 1 breath.
- Complete 20 cycles of 5 compressions and 1 breath (takes about 1 minute), then check the pulse. If you are alone, activate the EMS. If there is no pulse, restart CPR with chest compressions. Recheck the pulse every few minutes. If there is a pulse, give rescue breathing.
- Give CPR until:
  Infant revives.

OR

  Trained help, such as emergency medical technicians (EMTs), arrives and relieves you.

OR

  You are completely exhausted.

If infant is conscious and cannot cough, cry, or breathe . . .

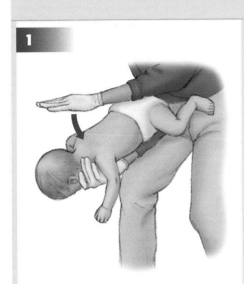

1

Give up to 5 back blows

- Hold infant's head and neck with 1 hand by firmly supporting infant's jaw between your thumb and fingers.
- Lay infant face down over your forearm with head lower than his or her chest. Brace your forearm and infant against your thigh.
- Give up to 5 distinct and separate back blows between shoulder blades with the heel of your hand.

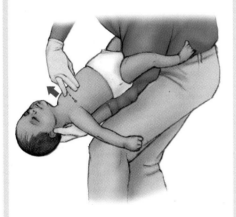

2

Give up to 5 chest thrusts

- Support the back of infant's head.
- Sandwich infant between your hands and arms, turn on back, with head lower than chest. If you are small, you may need to support infant on your lap.
- Imagine a line connecting infant's nipples.
- Place 3 fingers on sternum with your ring finger next to imaginary nipple line on the infant's feet side.
- Lift your ring finger off chest. If you feel the notch at the end of the sternum, move your fingers up a little.
- Give up to 5 separate and distinct thrusts with index and middle fingers on sternum in a manner similar to CPR chest compressions, but at a slower rate.
- Keep fingers in contact with chest between chest thrusts.

3

Repeat

- Give up to 5 back blows, then
- Give up to 5 chest thrusts until infant becomes unconscious.

OR

Object is expelled, and infant begins to breathe or cough forcefully.

If infant is motionless . . .

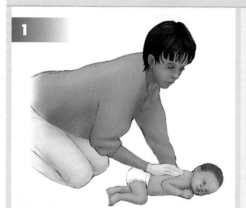

Check responsiveness
- If spine injury is suspected, move infant only if absolutely necessary.
- Tap infant's shoulder.

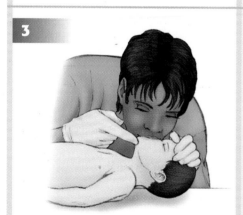

Send bystander, if available, to activate EMS. If you are alone, resuscitate for 1 minute before activating EMS.

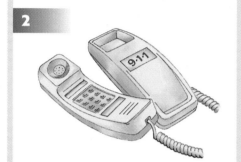

Give 2 slow breaths
- Open the airway with head-tilt/chin-lift.
- Seal your mouth over infant's mouth and nose.
- Give 2 slow breaths (1 to 1½ seconds each).

If first breath did not go in, retilt the head and try 1 more slow breath.

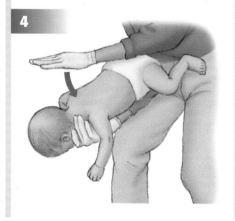

Give up to 5 back blows
- Hold infant's head and neck with 1 hand by firmly supporting infant's jaw between your thumb and fingers.
- Lay infant face down over your forearm with head lower than chest. Brace your forearm and infant against your thigh.
- Give up to 5 distinct and separate back blows between shoulder blades with the heel of your hand.

5

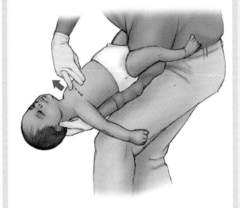

Give up to 5 chest thrusts

- Support the back of infant's head.
- Sandwich infant between your hands and arms, then turn infant on back, with head lower than chest. If you are small, you may need to support infant on your lap.
- Imagine a line connecting infant's nipples.
- Place 3 fingers on sternum with your ring finger next to imaginary nipple line on the infant's feet side.
- Lift your ring finger off chest. If you feel the notch at the end of the sternum, move your fingers up a little.
- Give up to 5 separate and distinct thrusts with index and middle fingers on sternum in a manner similar to CPR chest compressions but at a slower rate.
- Keep fingers in contact with chest between chest thrusts.

6

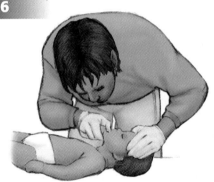

Check mouth for foreign object

- Grasp both tongue and jaw between your thumb and fingers and lift up.
- If object is visible, remove it with a finger sweep by sliding your little finger of the other hand alongside cheek to base of tongue using a hooking action.
- Do *not* try to remove an object you cannot see (a "blind finger sweep").
- Do not push object deeper.

7

Repeat

1. Give 1 slow breath.
2. Give up to 5 back blows.
3. Give up to 5 chest thrusts.
4. Check mouth for foreign object. If object is visible, use finger sweep.

Repeat until object is expelled or EMS arrives. If you are alone and after 1 minute the object has not been expelled, take infant with you and call the EMS.

Two-Rescuer CPR Procedures

(Laypersons should learn only one-rescuer CPR. Professional rescuers such as EMTs and other health care professionals should learn both one-rescuer and two-rescuer CPR.)

Entry of second rescuer when one-person CPR is in progress	#1 is performing one-rescuer CPR
	#2 says:
	• "I know CPR."
	• "EMS has been activated."
	• "Can I help?"
	#1 • completes CPR cycle (15 compressions and ends on 2 breaths)
	• says, "Take over compressions."
	• checks pulse and breathing (5 seconds)
	• if pulse absent, says, "No pulse, continue CPR."
	#2 • gives 5 compressions (at rate of 80–100 per minute)
	• after every 5th compression, pauses for #1 rescuer to give 1 full breath
	#1 • monitors victim while #2 performs compressions:
	   (a) watches chest rise during breaths
	   (b) feels carotid pulse during compressions
	• gives 1 full breath after every 5th compression given by #2 rescuer

Two rescuers starting CPR at the same time	#1 (ventilator) • assesses victim; if no breaths, gives 2 slow breaths; if no pulse, tells #2 to start compressions • gives 1 full breath after every 5th compression given by #2 #2 (compressor) • finds hand position and gets ready to give compressions • gives 5 compressions after #1 says to start them • pauses after every 5th compression for #1 to give 1 full breath
Switching during two-rescuer CPR	#2 (compressor) • signals when to change by saying, "Change and, two and, three and, four and, five" or "Change on the next breath." • after #1 gives breath, #2 moves to victim's head and completes pulse and breathing check (5 seconds); if pulse is absent, says, "No pulse, begin CPR." • gives a full breath after every cycle of 5 compressions #1 (ventilator) • gives 1 full breath at the end of 5th compression and moves to victim's chest • finds hand position and gets ready to give compressions • begins cycles of 5 compressions after every breath
How an untrained rescuer can help	• goes for help • monitors pulse and breathing, with some direction • gives CPR with directions (can learn compressions easier with trained rescuer giving breaths)

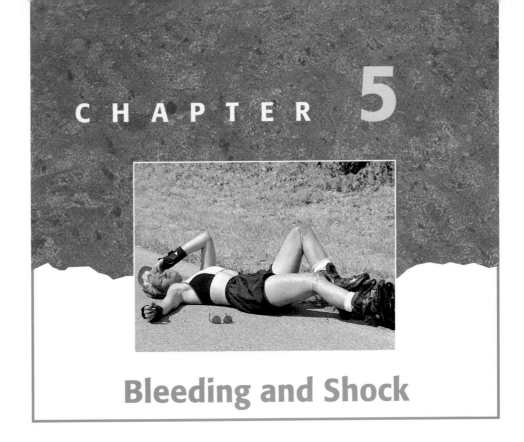

C H A P T E R 5

Bleeding and Shock

Bleeding

External Bleeding

External bleeding occurs when blood can be seen coming from an open wound. The term hemorrhage refers to a large amount of bleeding in a short time.

Types of External Bleeding

External bleeding can be classified into three types according to its source. In arterial bleeding, blood spurts (up to several feet) from the wound. Arterial bleeding is the most serious type of bleeding because blood is lost at a fast rate, leading to a large blood loss. Arterial bleeding also is less likely to clot because blood can clot only when it is flowing slowly or not at all. However, unless a very large artery has been cut, it is unlikely that a person will bleed to death before the flow can be controlled. Nevertheless, arterial bleeding is dangerous, and some external means of control must be used to stop it.

In venous bleeding, blood from a vein flows steadily or gushes. Venous bleeding is easier to control than arterial bleeding. Most veins collapse when cut. Bleeding from deep veins, however, can be as massive and as hard to control as arterial bleeding.

In capillary bleeding, blood oozes from capillaries. The most common type of bleeding, capillary bleeding usually is not serious and is controlled easily. Quite often, this type of bleeding will clot off by itself.

What to Do

Regardless of the type of bleeding or the type of wound, first aid is the same. First, and most important, you must control the bleeding:

1. Protect yourself against disease by wearing latex gloves. If latex gloves are not available, use several layers of gauze pads, plastic wrap, a plastic bag,

SKILL SCAN: Bleeding Control

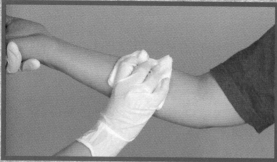

1.

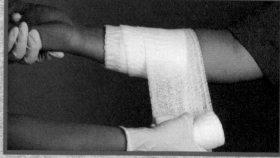

2.

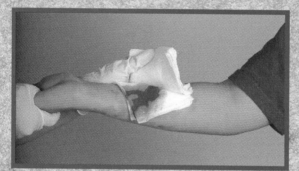

3.

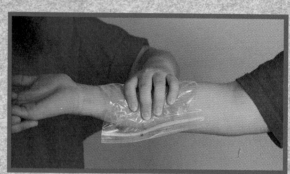

4.

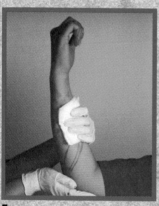

5.

1. Direct pressure stops most bleeding. Wearing disposable gloves, place sterile gauze pad or clean cloth over wound. If bleeding does not stop in 10 minutes, press harder over a wider area.

2. A pressure bandage can free you to attend to other injuries or victims.

3. Do not remove a blood-soaked dressing. Add more on top.

4. If disposable gloves are not available, use another barrier or extra gauze pads or cloths.

5. If bleeding persists, use elevation to help reduce blood flow. Combine with direct pressure over the wound.

6. If bleeding still continues, apply pressure at a pressure point to slow blood flow. Locations are: **(a)** brachial or **(b)** femoral. Use with direct pressure over the wound.

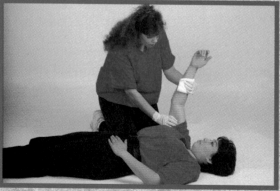

6a.

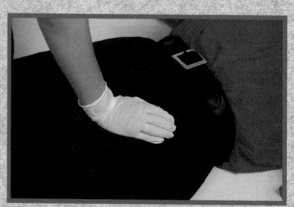

6b.

or waterproof material. You can even have the victim apply pressure with his or her own hand.

2. Expose the wound by removing or cutting the clothing to see where the blood is coming from.

 CAUTION: DO NOT

- touch a wound with your bare hands. If you must use your bare hands, do so only as a last resort. After the bleeding has stopped and the wound has been cared for, vigorously wash your hands with soap and water.
- use direct pressure on an eye injury, a wound with an embedded object, or a skull fracture.
- remove a blood-soaked dressing. Apply another dressing on top and keep pressing.

3. Place a sterile gauze pad or a clean cloth (e.g., handkerchief, washcloth, or towel) over the entire wound and apply direct pressure with your fingers or the palm of your hand. The gauze or cloth allows you to apply even pressure. Direct pressure stops most bleeding. Be sure the pressure remains constant, is not too light, and is applied to the bleeding source. Do not remove blood-soaked dressings; simply apply new dressings over the old ones.

4. If bleeding does not stop in 10 minutes, the pressure may be too light or in the wrong location. Press harder over a wider area for another 10 minutes. If the bleeding is from an arm or leg, while still applying pressure, elevate the injured area above heart level to reduce blood flow. Elevation allows gravity to make it difficult for the body to pump blood to the affected extremity. Elevation alone, however, will not stop bleeding and must be used in combination with direct pressure over the wound.

5. If the bleeding continues, apply pressure at a pressure point to slow the flow of blood, in combination with direct pressure over the wound. A pressure point is where an artery is near the skin's surface and where it passes close to a bone, against which it can be compressed. Two pressure points on both sides of the body are the most accessible: the brachial point in the upper inside arm and the femoral point in the groin. Using pressure points requires skill, and

unless the exact location of the pulse point is used, the pressure-point technique is useless. Most bleeding, however, is stopped by direct pressure over the wound.

6. After the bleeding stops or to free you to attend to other injuries or victims, use a pressure bandage to hold the dressing on the wound. Wrap a roller gauze bandage tightly over the dressing and above and below the wound site.

 CAUTION: DO NOT

- apply a pressure bandage so tight that it cuts off circulation. Check the radial pulse if the bandage is on an arm; for a leg, check the pulse between the inside ankle bone knob and the Achilles tendon (posterior tibial).
- use a tourniquet. They are rarely needed and can damage nerves and blood vessels. Use of a tourniquet may cause the loss of an arm or leg. If you do use one, apply wide, flat materials—never rope or wire—and do not loosen it. Remember: Use of a tourniquet usually means the extremity will have to be amputated.

7. When direct pressure cannot be applied (e.g., in the case of a protruding bone, skull fracture, or embedded object) use a doughnut-shaped (ring) pad to control bleeding. To make a ring pad, wrap one end of a narrow bandage (roller or cravat) several times around your four fingers to form a loop. Pass the other end of the bandage through the loop and wrap it around and around until the entire bandage is used and a ring has been made.

Internal Bleeding

Internal bleeding occurs when the skin is unbroken and blood is not visible. It can be difficult to detect and can be life threatening. Internal bleeding comes from injuries that do not break the skin or from nontraumatic disorders such as ulcers.

What to Look For

The signs of internal bleeding may take days to appear:

BLEEDING

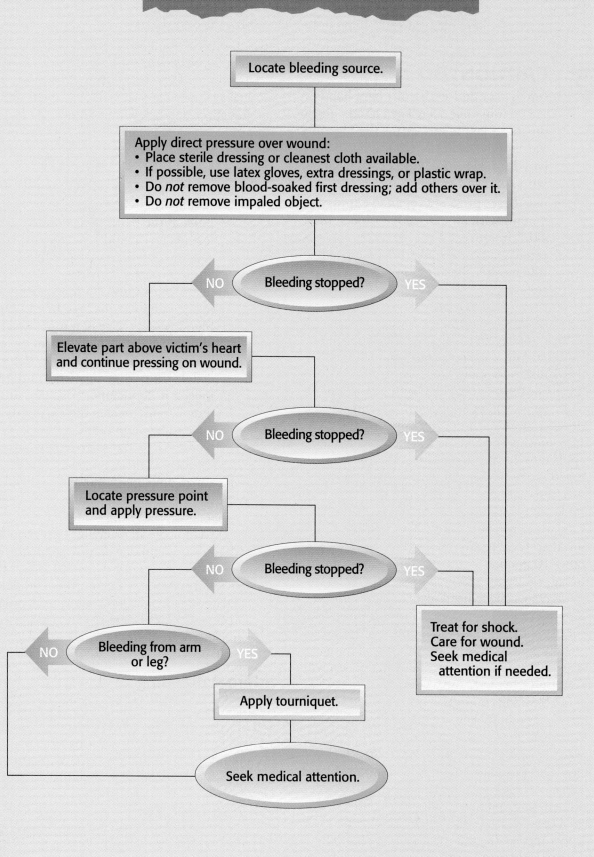

Locate bleeding source.

Apply direct pressure over wound:
- Place sterile dressing or cleanest cloth available.
- If possible, use latex gloves, extra dressings, or plastic wrap.
- Do *not* remove blood-soaked first dressing; add others over it.
- Do *not* remove impaled object.

Bleeding stopped? — NO / YES

Elevate part above victim's heart and continue pressing on wound.

Bleeding stopped? — NO / YES

Locate pressure point and apply pressure.

Bleeding stopped? — NO / YES

Bleeding from arm or leg? — NO / YES

Apply tourniquet.

Treat for shock.
Care for wound.
Seek medical attention if needed.

Seek medical attention.

- bruises or contusions of the skin
- painful, tender, rigid, bruised abdomen
- fractured ribs or bruises on chest
- vomiting or coughing up blood
- stools that are black or contain bright red blood

What to Do

For severe internal bleeding, follow these steps:

1. Monitor the ABCDs.
2. Expect vomiting. If vomiting occurs, keep the victim lying on his or her left side for drainage, to prevent inhalation of vomitus, and to prevent expulsion of vomit from the stomach.
3. Treat for shock by raising the victim's legs 8–12 inches and cover the victim with a coat or blanket to keep warm. See page 44 for when to use other body positions.
4. Seek immediate medical attention.

 CAUTION: DO NOT
- **give a victim anything to eat or drink. It could cause nausea and vomiting, which could result in aspiration. It could cause complications if surgery is needed.**

Bruises are a form of internal bleeding but are not life threatening. To treat bruises see page 99.

Shock

Shock refers to circulatory system failure, which happens when oxygenated blood is not provided in sufficient amounts for every body part. Because every injury affects the circulatory system to some degree, first aiders should automatically treat injured victims for shock.

To understand shock, think of the circulatory system as having three components: a working pump (the heart), a network of pipes (the blood vessels), and an adequate amount of fluid (the blood) pumped through the pipes. Damage to any of those components can deprive tissues of blood and produce the condition known as shock.

Shock can be classified as one of three types according to which component has failed.

- *Pump failure:* failure of the heart to pump sufficient blood. For example, a major heart attack can cause damage to the heart muscle so the heart cannot squeeze and therefore cannot push blood through the blood vessels.
- *Fluid loss:* loss of a significant amount of fluid from the system, usually blood.
- *Pipe failure:* blood vessels (pipes) enlarge and the blood supply is insufficient to fill them. Results when the nervous system is damaged (e.g., spinal cord is damaged or victim has overdosed on drugs).

What to Look For

- altered mental status: anxiety and restlessness
- pale, cold, and clammy skin, lips, and nail beds
- nausea and vomiting
- breathing and pulse rapid
- unresponsiveness when shock is severe

What to Do

Even if an injured victim does not have signs or symptoms of shock, first aiders should treat for shock.

1. Treat life-threatening injuries and other severe injuries.
2. Lay the victim on his or her back.

 CAUTION: DO NOT
- **raise the legs of victims with head injuries or strokes. Slightly raise the victim's head if no spine injury is suspected.**
- **place victims with breathing difficulties, chest injuries, penetrating eye injuries, or heart attack on their backs. Place them in a half-sitting position to help breathing.**
- **place victims rated as V, P, or U (see page 15) or vomiting victims on their backs. Use the recovery position (see page 22). If a spine injury is suspected, do *not* move the victim.**
- **place an advanced (third trimester) pregnant woman on her back—instead, place her on her left side to avoid pressing the vena cava.**

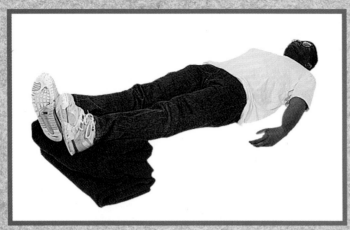

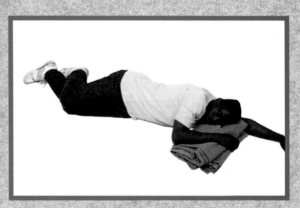

1. Usual shock position. Elevate the legs 8–12 inches. Do not lift the foot of bed or stretcher.
EXCEPTIONS:
2. Elevate the head for injuries or stroke.
3. Lay an unconscious, unresponsive, or vomiting victim on his or her left side.
4. Use a half-sitting position for those with breathing difficulties, chest injuries, or a heart attack.
5. Keep victim flat if a neck or spine injury is suspected or victim has leg fractures.

1.

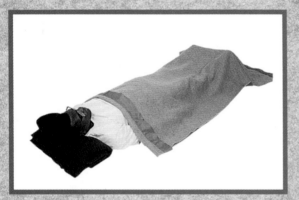

2.

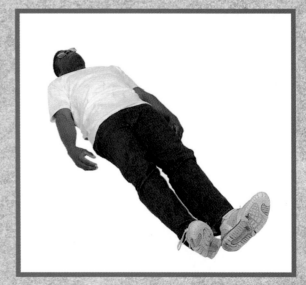

3.

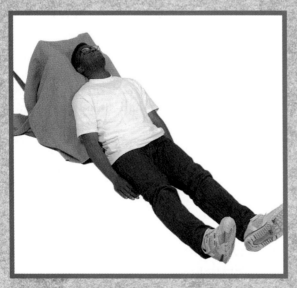

4.

5.

3. Raise the victim's legs 8–12 inches. Raising the legs allows the blood to drain from the legs back to the heart.
4. Prevent body heat loss by putting blankets and coats under and over the victim.

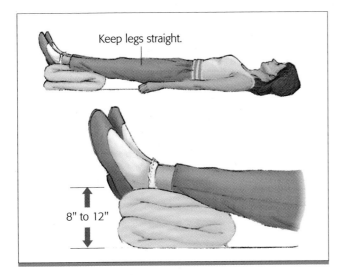
Keep legs straight.

8" to 12"

Elevate the legs to circulate blood to the vital organs.

 CAUTION: DO NOT

- **raise the legs more than 12 inches since that would affect the victim's breathing by having the abdominal organs push up against the diaphragm.**
- **lift the foot of a bed or stretcher— breathing will be affected, and the blood flow from the brain may be retarded and lead to brain swelling.**
- **raise the legs of a victim with head injuries, stroke, chest injuries, breathing difficulty, unconsciousness. Place the victim in the proper position, as described above.**

 CAUTION: DO NOT

- **try to warm the victim.**
- **give the victim anything to eat or drink. It could cause nausea and vomiting, which could result in aspiration. It could also cause complications if surgery is needed. Sucking on a clean cloth soaked in water will relieve a victim's dry mouth.**

Anaphylaxis

A powerful reaction to substances eaten or injected can occur within minutes or even seconds. This reaction, called **anaphylaxis**, can cause death if it is not treated immediately.

Common Causes of Anaphylaxis

Like less severe allergic reactions, anaphylaxis is an abnormal response that doesn't bother most people but causes symptoms in those who have a hypersensitivity. Well-known causes of anaphylaxis include:

- medications (penicillin and related drugs, aspirin, sulfa drugs)
- food and food additives (shellfish, nuts, eggs, monosodium glutamate, nitrates, nitrites)
- insect stings (honeybee, yellow jacket, wasp, hornet, fire ant)
- plant pollen
- radiographic dyes

What to Look For

Anaphylaxis typically comes on within minutes of exposure to the offending substance, peaks in 15 to 30 minutes, and is over within hours.

Signs and symptoms of anaphylaxis include:

- sneezing, coughing, wheezing
- shortness of breath
- tightness and swelling in the throat
- tightness in the chest
- increased pulse rate
- swelling of the mucous membranes (tongue, mouth, nose)
- blueness around lips and mouth
- dizziness
- nausea and vomiting

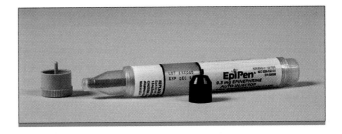
Doctor-prescribed preloaded epinephrine autoinjector

CAUTION: DO NOT

- mistake anaphylaxis for other reactions such as hyperventilation, anxiety attacks, alcohol intoxication, or low blood sugar.

What to Do

1. Check the ABCs.
2. Seek immediate medical attention.
3. If the victim has his or her own physician prescribed epinephrine, help the victim use it.

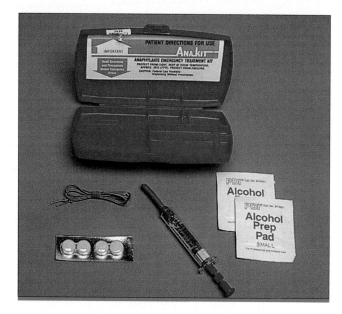

Doctor-prescribed preloaded epinephrine with 2 shots

LEARNING ACTIVITIES 5

Bleeding

Directions: Circle Yes if you agree with the statement, and circle No if you disagree.

Yes   No   1. Most cases of bleeding require more than direct pressure for it to stop.

Yes   No   2. Remove and replace blood-soaked dressings.

Yes   No   3. Elevating an arm or leg alone will not control bleeding and must be used in combination with direct pressure over the wound.

Yes   No   4. If direct pressure and elevation fail to control bleeding, the next step would be to use a tourniquet.

Yes   No   5. Tourniquets are often needed.

Scenario: Jim, a 25-year-old construction worker, has been badly cut on his thigh by a circular power saw. Blood is flowing heavily. The cut is about six to eight inches long. What should you do?

_____

_____

_____

Shock

Yes   No   1. Most severely injured victims should have their legs raised.

Yes   No   2. Give the victim something to drink.

Yes   No   3. Prevent body heat loss by putting blankets under and over the victim.

Yes   No   4. A shock victim with head injuries should be placed on his or her side.

Yes   No   5. A shock victim with breathing difficulty or chest injury should be placed on his or her back with the legs raised.

Scenario: You have controlled the construction worker's bleeding. He appears to be pale and is anxious and restless. What should you do?

_____

_____

_____

Anaphylaxis

Yes   No   1. Anaphylaxis is another form of fainting.

Yes   No   2. Anaphylaxis can kill.

Yes   No   3. Ask the victim if he or she has doctor-prescribed epinephrine.

Scenario: On a nice summer day, Susan is weeding in the front of the company's office building. All of a sudden, she begins slapping her legs. She has disturbed a nest of yellow jackets, which proceed to sting her more than a dozen times. Susan complains that she feels hot, and has begun coughing, sneezing, and wheezing. You notice that her face seems to be getting puffy. What should you do?

_____

_____

_____

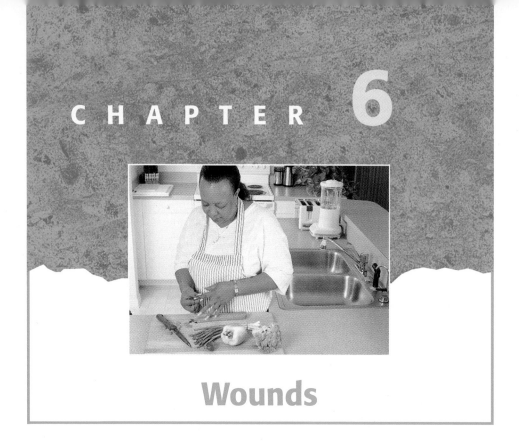

CHAPTER 6

Wounds

Open Wounds

An open wound is a break in the skin's surface in which there is external bleeding. Victims of open wounds are susceptible to blood loss and infection.

There are several types of open wounds. With an abrasion, the top layer of skin is removed, with little or no blood loss. Abrasions tend to be painful, because the nerve endings often are abraded along with the skin. Ground-in debris may be present. This type of wound can be serious if it covers a large area or if foreign matter becomes embedded in it. An abrasion is also known as a "scrape," "road rash," and "rug burn."

A laceration is cut skin with jagged, irregular edges. This type of wound is usually caused by a forceful tearing away of skin tissue.

Incisions tend to be smooth edged, resembling a surgical cut or a paper cut. The amount of bleeding depends on the depth, the location, and the size of the wound.

Punctures are usually deep, narrow wounds in the skin and underlying organs. An example is a stab wound from a nail or a knife. The entrance is usually small, and the risk of infection is high. The object causing the injury may remain impaled in the wound.

With an avulsion, a flap of skin is torn loose and is either hanging from the body or completely removed. This type of wound can bleed heavily. If the flap is still attached and folded back, lay it flat and realign it into its normal position. Avulsions most often involve ears, fingers, and hands.

An amputation involves the cutting or tearing off of a body part, such as a finger, toe, hand, foot, arm, or leg.

What to Do

1. Protect yourself against disease by wearing latex gloves. If latex gloves are not available, use several layers of gauze pads, plastic wrap or bags, or

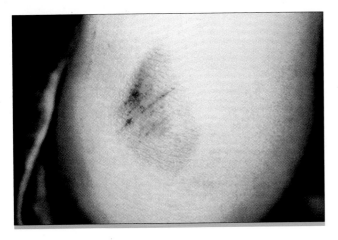

Abrasion

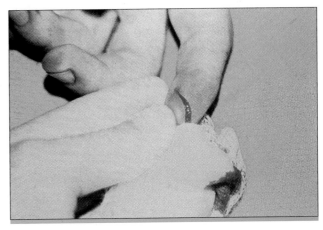

Laceration

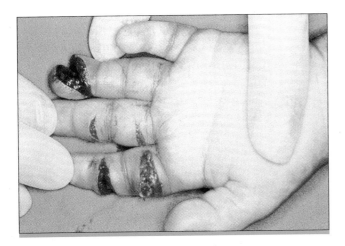

Incision

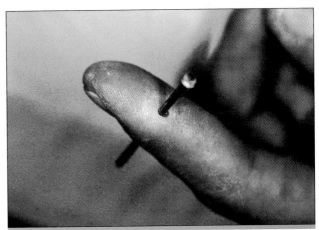

Puncture

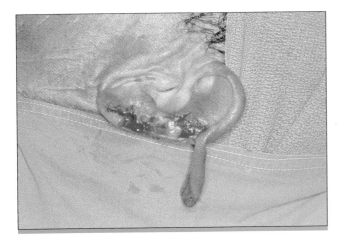

Avulsion

waterproof material. You can even have the victim apply pressure with his or her own hand. Your bare hand should be used *only* as a last resort.

2. Expose the wound by removing or cutting the clothing to see where the blood is coming from.
3. Control bleeding by using direct pressure and, if needed, the other methods described in Chapter 5.

Cleaning a Wound

A victim's wound should be cleaned to help prevent infection. Wound cleaning may restart bleeding, but it should be done anyway. For severe bleeding, leave the pressure bandage in place until you are certain that bleeding has stopped.

1. Scrub your hands vigorously with soap and water. Then, if they are available, put on latex gloves.
2. Clean the wound.
   For a shallow wound (e.g., laceration, incision):
   • Wash inside it with soap and water.

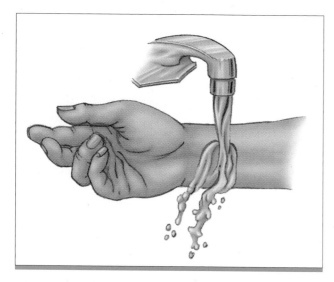

Irrigate a wound with water under pressure.

- Irrigate the wound with water (use water that is clean enough to drink). Run water directly into the wound and allow it to run out. Irrigation with water needs pressure (minimum 5 to 8 psi) for adequate tissue cleansing. Water from a faucet provides the pressure and the amount needed. Pouring the water or using a bulb syringe is not forceful enough.

For a wound with a high risk for infection (e.g., an animal bite, a very dirty or ragged wound, a puncture), seek medical attention for wound cleaning unless you are in a remote setting (greater than one hour from medical attention). In this case, clean the wound as best you can.

3. With sterile tweezers, remove small objects not flushed out by irrigation. A dirty abrasion or other wound that is not cleaned will leave a "tattoo" on the victim's skin.

 CAUTION: DO NOT

- clean large, extremely dirty, or life-threatening wounds. Let hospital emergency department personnel do the cleaning.
- scrub a wound. Scrubbing a wound is debatable, and it can bruise the tissue.

4. Cover the wound with a sterile and, if possible, nonstick dressing. Keep the dressing clean and dry. To keep the dressing in place on an arm or leg, use a self-adhering roller bandage or tape; on other parts of the body, tape the four sides of the dressing onto the skin. For a shallow wound, an antibiotic ointment can be applied.

5. Change the dressing daily, more often if it gets wet or dirty.

 CAUTION: DO NOT

- irrigate a wound with full-strength iodine preparations (e.g., Betadine 10%) or isopropyl alcohol (70%). They kill body cells as well as bacteria and are painful. Also, some people are allergic to iodine.
- use hydrogen peroxide. It does not kill bacteria, and it adversely affects capillary blood flow and wound healing.
- use antibiotic ointment on wounds that require sutures or on puncture wounds (the ointment may prevent drainage). Use an antibiotic ointment only on abrasions and shallow wounds.
- soak a wound to clean it. No evidence supports the effectiveness of soaking.
- close the wound with tape (e.g., butterfly tape, Steri-strips). Infection is more likely when bacteria are trapped in the wound. An extremity (e.g., hand, foot) wound can be sutured within 6 to 8 hours of the injury. Suturing of a head or trunk wound can wait up to 24 hours after the injury. Some wounds can be sutured 3 to 5 days after the injury.
- breathe on a wound or the dressing.

Covering a Wound

For a small wound that does not require sutures, cover it with a thin layer of antibiotic ointment (e.g., Neosporin or Polysporin). Such ointments can kill a great many bacteria and rarely cause allergic reactions. They are available without prescription.

Cover the wound with a sterile dressing. Do not close the wound with tape (butterflies). Bacteria may remain, leading to a greater chance of infection than if the wound were left open and covered by a sterile dressing. Closing a wound should be left to a physician.

Dressings and bandages are two different kinds of first aid supplies. A dressing is applied over a wound to control bleeding and prevent contamination. A bandage holds the dressing in place. Dressings should be sterile or as clean as possible; bandages need not be.

If a wound bleeds after a dressing has been applied and the dressing becomes stuck, leave it on as long as the wound is healing. Pulling the scab loose to change the dressing retards healing and increases the chance of infection. If a dressing must be removed, soak it in warm water to help soften the scab and make removal easier.

Wound Infection

Any wound, large or small, can become infected. Once an infection begins, damage can be extensive, so prevention is the best way to avoid the problem. A wound should be cleaned using the procedures described above.

It is important to know how to recognize and treat an infected wound. Most infected wounds swell and become reddened. They may give a sensation of warmth and develop a throbbing pain and a pus discharge. The victim may develop a fever and swelling of the lymph nodes. One or more red streaks may appear, leading from the wound toward the heart. This is a serious sign that the infection is spreading and could cause death. If chills and fever develop, the infection has reached the circulatory system (known as blood poisoning). Seek medical attention immediately.

Tetanus

The tetanus bacterium by itself does not cause tetanus. But when it enters a wound that contains little oxygen (e.g., a puncture wound), the bacterium can produce a toxin, which is a powerful poison. The toxin travels through the nervous system to the brain and the spinal cord. It then causes contractions of certain muscle groups (particularly in the jaw). There is no known antidote to the toxin once it enters the nervous system.

A vaccination can completely prevent tetanus. Everyone needs an initial series of vaccinations to prepare the immune system to defend against the toxin. Then a booster shot once every 5 to 10 years is sufficient to jog the immune system's memory.

The guidelines for tetanus immunization boosters are as follows:

- Anyone with a wound who has never been immunized against tetanus should be given a tetanus vaccine and booster immediately.
- A victim who was once immunized but has not received a tetanus booster within the last 10 years should receive a booster.
- A victim with a dirty wound who has not had a booster for over 5 years should receive a booster.
- Tetanus immunization shots must be given within 72 hours of the injury to be effective.

Amputations
What to Do

1. Control the bleeding with direct pressure and elevate the extremity. Apply a dry dressing or bulky cloths. Be sure to protect yourself against disease. Tourniquets are rarely needed and if used will destroy tissue, blood vessels, and nerves necessary for replantation.
2. Treat the victim for shock.
3. Recover the amputated part and, whenever possible, take it with the victim. However, in multi-casualty cases, in reduced lighting conditions, or when untrained people transport the victim, someone may be requested to locate and take the severed body part to the hospital after the victim's departure.
4. To care for the amputated body part:
   - If possible, rinse it with clean water to remove any debris; do not scrub. The amputated portion does not need to be cleaned.
   - Wrap the amputated part with a dry sterile gauze or other clean cloth.
   - Put the wrapped amputated part in a plastic bag or other waterproof container (e.g., a cup or glass).
   - Place the bag or container with the wrapped part on a bed of ice.
5. Seek medical attention immediately.

Amputated body parts left uncooled for more than 6 hours have little chance of survival; 18 hours is probably the maximum time allowable for a part that has been cooled properly. Muscles without blood lose viability within 4 to 6 hours.

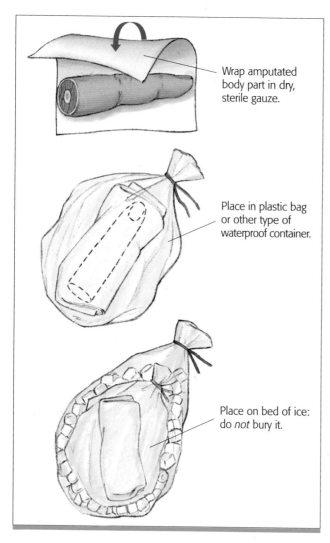

Wrap amputated body part in dry, sterile gauze.

Place in plastic bag or other type of waterproof container.

Place on bed of ice: do *not* bury it.

Care of an amputated part

 CAUTION: DO NOT

- try to decide whether a body part is salvageable or too small to save—leave the decision to a physician.
- wrap an amputated part in a wet dressing or cloth. Using a wet wrap on the part can cause waterlogging and tissue softening, which will make reattachment more difficult.
- bury an amputated part in ice—place it *on* ice. Reattaching frostbitten parts is usually unsuccessful.
- use dry ice.

- cut a skin "bridge," a tendon, or other structure that is connecting a partially attached part to the rest of the body. Reposition the part in the normal position, wrap the part in a dry sterile dressing or clean cloth, and place an ice pack on it.

Impaled Objects

What to Do

1. Do not remove or move an impaled object. Movement of any kind could produce additional bleeding and tissue damage.
2. Expose the area. Remove or cut away any clothing surrounding the injury. If clothes cover the object, leave them in place; removing them could cause the object to move.
3. Control any bleeding with direct pressure. Straddle the object with gauze. Do not press directly on the object or along the wound next to the cutting edge, especially if the object has sharp edges.
4. Stabilize the object. Secure a bulky dressing or clean cloth around the object. Some experts suggest securing 75 percent of the object with bulky dressing or cloths to reduce motion.
5. Shorten the object only if necessary. In most cases, do not shorten the object by cutting or breaking it. There are times, however, when cutting off or shortening the object allows for easier transportation. Be sure to stabilize the object before shortening it. Remember that the victim will feel any vibrations from the object being cut and that the injury could be worsened.

Closed Wounds

A closed wound happens when a blunt object strikes the body. The skin is not broken, but tissue and blood vessels beneath the skin's surface are crushed, causing bleeding within a confined area.

What to Do

1. Control bleeding by applying an ice pack for no more than 20 minutes.

2. Apply an elastic bandage with a gauze pad between the bandage and the skin.
3. Check for a possible fracture.
4. Elevate an injured extremity above the victim's heart level to decrease pain and swelling.

Wounds That Require Medical Attention

At some point, you probably will have to decide about obtaining medical assistance for a wounded victim. As a guideline, seek medical attention for the following conditions:

- arterial bleeding
- uncontrolled bleeding
- a deep incision, laceration, or avulsion that
  - goes into the muscle or bone
  - is located on a body part that bends (e.g., elbow or knee)
  - tends to gape widely
  - is located on the thumb or palm of the hand (nerves may be affected)
- a large or deep puncture wound
- a large embedded object or a deeply embedded object of any size
- foreign matter left in the wound
- human or animal bite
- possibility of a noticeable scar (sutured cuts usually heal with less scarring than unsutured ones)
- a wide, gaping wound
- an eyelid cut (to prevent later drooping)
- a slit lip (easily scarred)
- internal bleeding
- any wound you are not certain how to treat
- victim's immunization against tetanus not up to date

Sutures (Stitches)

If sutures are needed, they should be made by a physician within six to eight hours of the injury. Suturing wounds allows faster healing, reduces infection, and lessens scarring.

Some wounds do not usually require sutures:

- wounds in which the skin's cut edges tend to fall together
- cuts less than one inch long that are not deep

Rather than close a gaping wound with butterfly bandages, cover the wound with sterile gauze. Closing the wound might trap bacteria inside, resulting in an infection. In most cases, a physician can be reached in time for sutures to be made.

Wound Care

Directions: Circle Yes if you agree with the statement, and circle No if you disagree.

Yes   No   1. Wash shallow wounds with soapy water.

Yes   No   2. Irrigating a wound with water needs pressure.

Yes   No   3. Wounds with a high risk for infection (e.g., animal bites, dirty wounds) require medical attention for proper wound cleaning.

Yes   No   4. Antibiotic ointment can be applied to any wound.

Yes   No   5. Hydrogen peroxide works well on wounds.

Scenario: Nancy, a 23-year-old, while using a knife to open a cardboard box lost her grip on the knife and received a shallow incision wound on her hand. What should you do?

_____

_____

_____

Amputations

Yes   No   1. Recover any amputated part, regardless of size, and take it with the victim to the nearest hospital.

Yes   No   2. Cut off a partially attached part.

Yes   No   3. Wrap an amputated part in a dry, sterile gauze dressing, enclose it in something waterproof, and keep it cool.

Yes   No   4. Keep an amputated part packed (buried) in ice.

Yes   No   5. Do NOT let an amputated part become "water-logged" since it makes reattaching more difficult.

Scenario: Matt is mowing long wet grass, which begins to back up at his mower's discharge opening. He reaches into the discharge chute to try to brush away a clump of grass, and his fingers are struck by the mower's blade. Two fingers are cut off. You find sitting on the ground firmly holding what remains of his fingers. What should you do?

_____

_____

_____

Impaled Objects

Yes   No   1. Removing an impaled object could cause more bleeding.

Yes   No   2. Prevent an impaled object from moving by placing bulky padding around the object.

Scenario: At a construction site, a 38-year-old worker drove a large nail through his left hand with a nail gun. What should you do?

_____

_____

_____

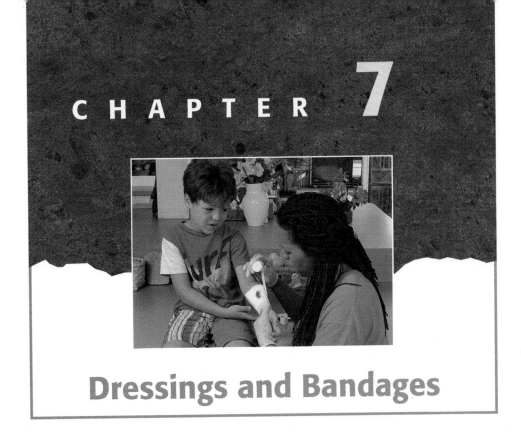

CHAPTER 7

Dressings and Bandages

Dressings

A dressing covers an open wound—it touches the wound. Whenever possible, a dressing should be:

- sterile. If a sterile dressing is not available, use a clean cloth (e.g., handkerchief, washcloth, towel)
- larger than the wound
- thick, soft, and compressible so pressure is evenly distributed over the wound
- lint free

  A dressing's purposes are to:
- control bleeding
- prevent infection and contamination
- absorb blood and wound drainage
- protect the wound from further injury

 CAUTION: DO NOT

- use fluffy cotton or cotton balls as a dressing. Cotton fibers can get in the wound and be difficult to remove.
- remove a blood-soaked dressing until the bleeding stops. Cover it with a new dressing.
- pull off a dressing stuck to a wound. If it needs to be removed, soak it off in warm water.

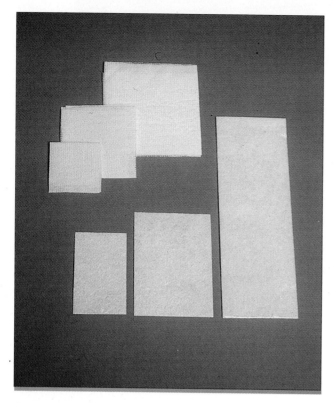

Gauze pads

Types of Dressings

- *Gauze pads* are used for small wounds. They come in separately wrapped packages of various sizes (e.g., 2 inch by 2 inch; 4 inch by 4 inch) and are sterile, unless the package is broken. Some gauze pads have a special coating to keep them from sticking to the wound and are especially helpful for burns or wounds secreting fluids.
- *Adhesive strips* (e.g., Band-Aids™) are used for small cuts and abrasions and are a combination of both a sterile dressing and a bandage.

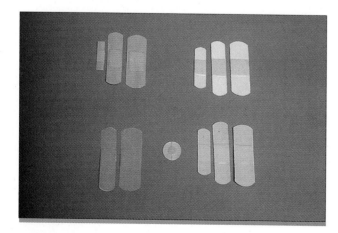

Adhesive strips

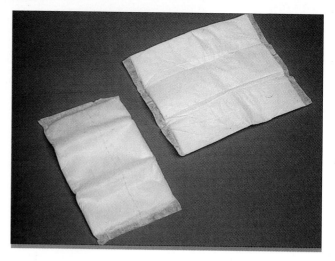

Trauma dressings

- *Trauma dressings* are made of large, thick, absorbent, sterile materials. Individually wrapped sanitary napkins can serve because of their bulk and absorbency, but they usually are not sterile.

Applying a Sterile Dressing
What to Do

1. If possible, wash your hands.
2. Use a dressing large enough to extend beyond the wound's edges. Hold the dressing by a corner. Place the dressing directly over the wound. Do not slide it on.
3. Cover the dressing with one of the types of bandages.

 CAUTION: DO NOT
- **touch any part of the wound or any part of the dressing that will be in contact with the wound.**
- **cough, breathe, or talk over the wound or dressing.**

Bandages

A bandage can be used to:

- hold a dressing in place over an open wound
- apply direct pressure over a dressing to control bleeding
- prevent or reduce swelling
- provide support and stability for an extremity or joint

A bandage should be clean but need not be sterile.

CAUTION: DO NOT

- apply a bandage directly over a wound. Put a sterile dressing on first.
- bandage so tightly as to restrict blood circulation. Always check the extremity's pulse. If you cannot feel the pulse, loosen the bandage.
- bandage so loosely that the dressing will slip. This is the most common bandaging error. Bandages tend to stretch after a short time.
- leave loose ends. They might get caught.
- cover fingers or toes unless they are injured. They need to be observed for color change should circulation be impaired.
- use elastic bandages over a wound. First aiders have a tendency to apply them too tightly.
- apply a circular bandage around a victim's neck—strangulation may occur.
- start a roller bandage above the wound. Instead, start below the wound and work upward.

Signs that a bandage is too tight:

- blue tinge of the fingernails or toenails
- blue or pale skin color
- tingling or loss of sensation
- coldness of the extremity
- inability to move the fingers or toes

Types of Bandages

There are four basic types of bandages:

- *Roller bandages* come in various widths, lengths, and types of material. For best results, use different widths for different body areas:
  - 1-inch width for fingers
  - 2-inch width for wrists, hands, feet
  - 3-inch width for ankles, elbows, arms
  - 4-inch width for knees, legs

Self-adhering, conforming bandages come as rolls of slightly elastic, gauzelike material in various widths. Their self-adherent quality makes them easy to use.

Gauze rollers are cotton, rigid, and nonelastic. They come in various widths (1, 2, and 3 inches) and usually are 10 yards long.

Elastic roller bandages are used for compression on sprains, strains, and contusions and

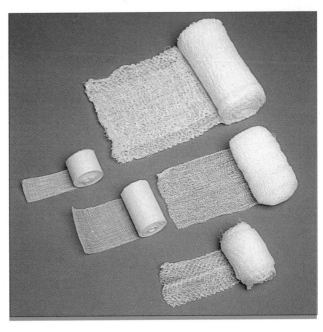

Self-adhering conforming bandages of various sizes

comes in various widths. Elastic bandages are not usually applied over dressings covering a wound.

When commercial roller bandages are unavailable, you can make *improvised bandages* from neckties or strips of cloth torn from a sheet or other similar material.

- *Triangular bandages* are available commercially or can be made from a 36- to 40-inch square of preshrunk cotton muslin material that is cut diagonally from corner to corner to produce two triangular pieces of cloth. The longest side is called the *base*; the corner directly across from the base is the *point*; the other two corners are called *ends*. A triangular bandage may be applied two ways:
  - Fully opened (not folded). Best used for an arm sling. When used to hold dressings in place, fully opened triangular bandages do not apply sufficient pressure on the wound.

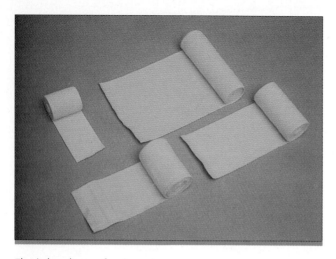

Elastic bandages of various sizes

- As a cravat (folded triangular). The point is folded to the center of the base and folded in

half again from the top to the base to form a cravat. It is used to hold splints in place, to apply pressure evenly over a dressing, or as a swathe (binder) around the victim's body to stabilize an injured arm in an arm sling.

- *Adhesive tape* comes in rolls and in a variety of widths. It is often used to secure roller bandages and small dressings in place. For those allergic to adhesive tape, use paper tape or special dermatologic tape.

- *Adhesive strips* are used for small cuts and abrasions and are a combination of a dressing and a bandage.

Roller Bandage for Hand: Method 1

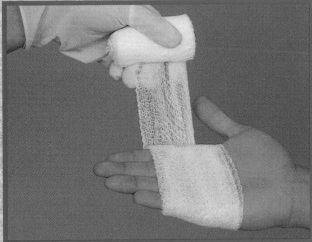

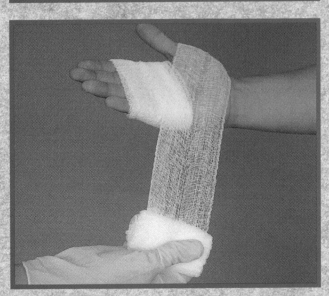

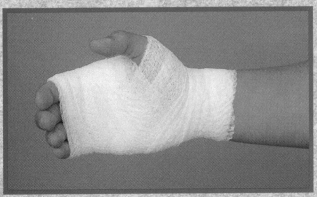

Roller Bandage for Hand: Method 2

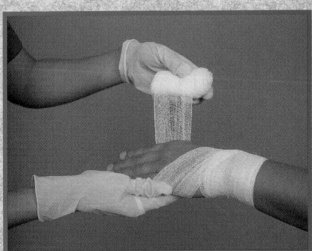

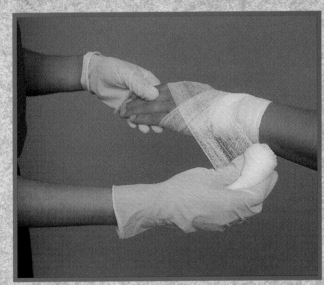

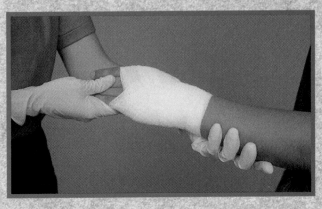

SKILL SCAN: Bandaging—Roller (Self-adhering), Figure-8

Roller Bandage for Elbow or Knee

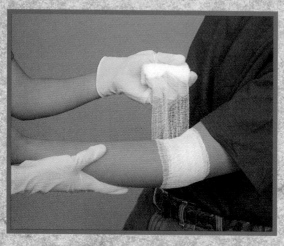

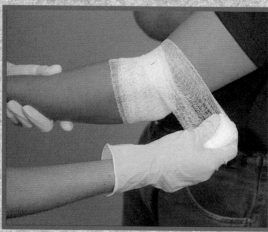

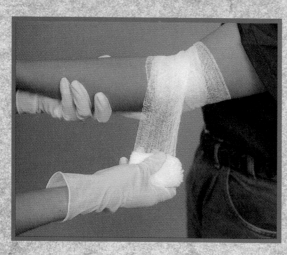

Roller Bandage for Ankle

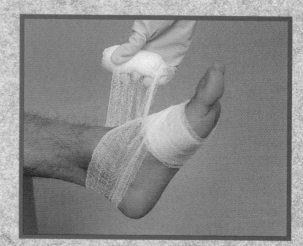

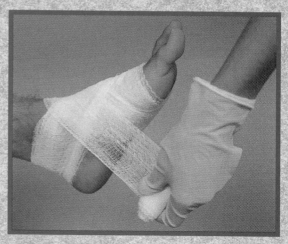

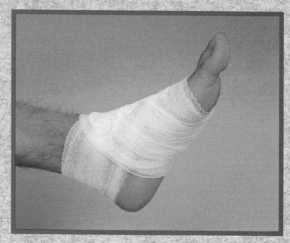

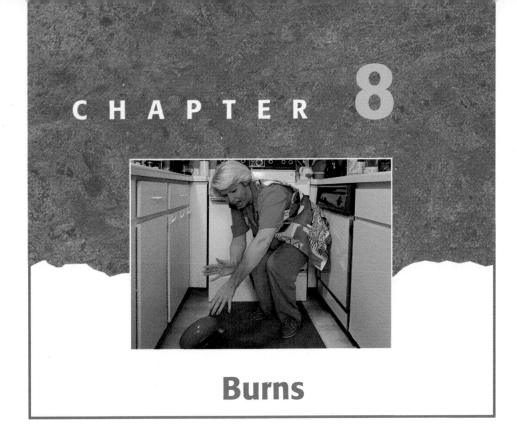

CHAPTER 8

Burns

Burn injuries can be classified as thermal (heat), chemical, or electrical.

- *Thermal burns*. Not all thermal burns are caused by flames. Contact with hot objects, flammable vapor that ignites and causes a flash or an explosion, and steam or hot liquid are other common causes of burns.
- *Chemical burns*. A wide range of chemical agents is capable of causing tissue damage and death on contact with the skin. As with thermal burns, the amount of tissue damage depends on the duration of contact, the skin thickness in the area of exposure, and the strength of the chemical agent. Chemicals will continue to cause tissue destruction until the chemical agent is removed. Three types of chemicals—acids, alkalis, and organic compounds—are responsible for most chemical burns.
- *Electrical burns*. The injury severity from exposure to electrical current depends on the type of current (direct or alternating), the voltage, the area of the body exposed, and the duration of contact.

Historically, burns have been described as *first-degree, second-degree,* and *third-degree* injuries. The terms *superficial, partial thickness,* and *full thickness* are often used by burn-care professionals because they are more descriptive of the tissue damage.

- First-degree (superficial) burns affect the skin's outer layer (epidermis). Characteristics include redness, mild swelling, tenderness, and pain. Healing occurs without scarring, usually within a week. The outer edges of deeper burns often are first-degree burns.
- Second-degree (partial-thickness) burns extend through the entire outer layer and into the inner skin layer. Blisters, swelling, weeping of fluids, and severe pain characterize these burns, which occur because the capil-

lary blood vessels in the dermis are damaged and give up fluid into surrounding tissues. Intact blisters provide a sterile waterproof covering. Once a blister breaks, a weeping wound results and infection risk increases.

- Third-degree (full-thickness) burns are severe burns that penetrate all the skin layers, into the underlying fat and muscle. The skin looks leathery, waxy, or pearly gray and sometimes charred. There is a dry appearance, because capillary blood vessels have been destroyed and no more fluid is brought to the area. The skin does not blanch after being pressed because the area is dead. The victim feels no pain from a third-degree burn because the nerve endings have been damaged or destroyed. Any pain that is felt is from surrounding burns of lesser degrees. A third-degree burn requires medical care, which involves removal of the dead tissue and often a skin graft to heal properly.

Respiratory damage may result from breathing heat or the products of combustion; from being burned by a flame while in a closed space; or from being in an explosion. Swelling results in 2 to 24 hours, restricting or even completely shutting off the airway so that air cannot reach the lungs. *All respiratory injuries must receive medical care.*

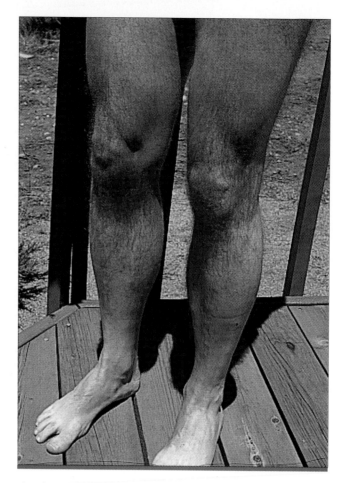

First-degree burn

Thermal Burns
What to Do

1. Stop the burning! Burns can continue to injure tissue for a surprisingly long time. If clothing has ignited, have the victim roll on the ground using the "stop, drop, and roll" method. Smother the flames with a blanket or douse the victim with water. Stop a person whose clothes are on fire from running; running only serves to fan the flames. Nor should the victim remain standing, because a standing victim is more apt to inhale flames. Once the fire is dead, remove all smoldering clothing; the burning may continue if the clothing is left on. Remove hot or burned clothing immediately.
2. Check the ABCs.
3. Determine the depth of the burn. It is difficult to tell a burn's depth because the destruction varies within the same burn. Even experienced physicians will not know the depth for several days after the burn. However, making an assess-

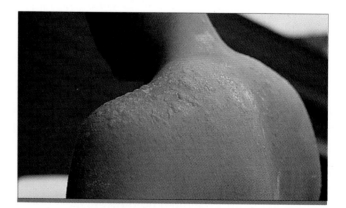

Second-degree burn blisters

ment of burn depth will help you decide whether to seek medical care for the victim.
4. Determine the extent of the burn. This means estimating how much body surface area the

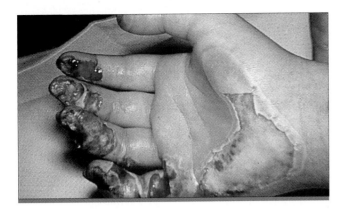
Second- and third-degree burns

quet effect on circulation and, in some cases, breathing. All these burns require medical care.

6. Determine if other injuries or preexisting medical problems exist or if the victim is elderly (over 55) or very young (under 5). A medical problem or belonging to one of those age groups increases a burn's severity.

7. Determine the burn's severity. This forms the basis for how to treat the burned victim. After you have evaluated the burn according to Steps 3 through 6, use the American Burn Association (ABA) guidelines to determine the burn's severity. Most burns are minor, occur at home, and can be managed outside a medical setting. Seek medical attention for all moderate and severe burns, as classified by the ABA, or if any of the following conditions applies:
   - The victim is under 5 or over 55 years of age.
   - The victim has difficulty breathing.
   - Other injuries exist.
   - An electrical injury exists.
   - The face, hands, feet, or genitals are burned.
   - Child abuse is suspected.
   - The surface area of a second-degree burn is greater than 15 percent of the body surface area.
   - The burn is third degree.

CAUTION: DO NOT
   - remove clothing stuck to the skin. Cut around the areas where clothing sticks to the skin.
   - pull on stuck clothing—pulling will further damage the skin.
   - forget to remove jewelry as soon as possible—swelling could make jewelry difficult to remove later.

burn covers. A rough guide known as the Rule of Nines assigns a percentage value to each part of an adult's body. The entire head is 9 percent, one complete arm is 9 percent, the front torso is 18 percent, the complete back is 18 percent, and each leg is 18 percent. The rule of nines must be modified to take into account the different proportions of a small child. In small children and infants, the head accounts for 18 percent and each leg is 14 percent.

For small or scattered burns, use the rule of the palm. The victim's hand, excluding the fingers and the thumb, represents about 1 percent of his or her total body surface. For a very large burn, estimate the *unburned* area in number of hands and subtract from 100 percent.

5. Determine what parts of the body are burned. Burns on the face, hands, feet, and genitals are more severe than on other body parts. A circumferential burn (one that goes around a finger, toe, arm, leg, neck, or chest) is considered more severe than a noncircumferential one because of the possible constriction and tourni-

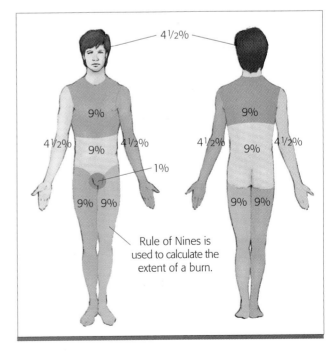
Rule of Nines

Table 8-1: Burn Severity

Minor Burns

First-degree burn covering < 50% BSA*

Second-degree burn covering <15% BSA in adults

Second-degree burn covering <10% BSA in children/ elderly persons

Third-degree burn covering <2% BSA

Moderate Burns

First-degree burn covering >50% BSA

Second-degree burn covering 15%–30% BSA in adults

Second-degree burn covering 10%–20% BSA in children/elderly persons

Third-degree burn covering <10% BSA

Critical Burns

Second-degree burn covering >30% BSA in adults

Second-degree burn covering >20% BSA in children/ elderly persons

Third-degree burn covering >10% BSA

Burns of hands, face, eyes, feet, or genitalia; also most inhalation injuries, electrical injuries, and burns accompanied by major trauma or significant preexisting conditions

*BSA = body surface area

Source: Adapted with permission from the American Burn Association categorization.

CAUTION: DO NOT

- apply cold to more than 20 percent of an adult's body surface (10 percent for children)—widespread cooling can cause hypothermia. Burn victims lose large amounts of heat and water.
- leave wet packs on wounds for long periods.
- use an ice pack unless it is the only source of cold. If you must use one, apply it for only 10–15 minutes, since frostbite and hypothermia can develop.
- apply salve, ointment, grease, butter, cream, spray, home remedy, or any other coating on a burn until it has been cooled. Such coatings are unsterile and can lead to infection. They also can seal in heat, causing further damage.

Burn Care

Burn care aims to reduce pain, protect against infection, and prevent evaporation.

Care of First-Degree Burns

1. Relieve pain by immersing the burned area in cold water or by applying a wet, cold cloth. Apply cold until the part is pain free both in and out of the water (usually in 10 minutes, but it may take up to 45 minutes). Cold also stops the burn's progression into deeper tissue. If cold water is unavailable, use any cold liquid you drink to reduce the burned skin's temperature.

2. Relieve pain and inflammation with aspirin or ibuprofen. Acetaminophen relieves pain but not inflammation.

3. Apply an aloe vera gel or an inexpensive moisturizer to keep the skin moistened and to avoid itching and peeling. Aloe vera has antimicrobial properties and is an effective analgesic.

CAUTION: DO NOT

- use a dressing. Most first-degree burns do not need a dressing.
- use anesthetic sprays because they may sensitize the skin to "-caine" anesthetics.

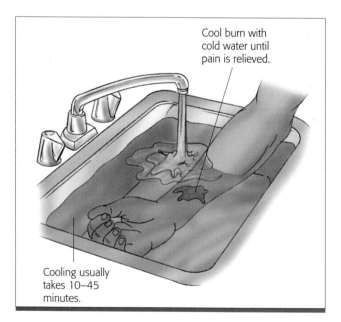

Cool burn with cold water until pain is relieved.

Cooling usually takes 10–45 minutes.

Immerse the burn in cold water.

Care of Second-Degree Burns

1. Relieve pain by immersing the burned area in cold water or by applying a wet, cold cloth. Apply cold until the part is pain free both in and out of the water (usually in 10 minutes, but it may take up to 45 minutes). Cold also stops the burn's progression into deeper tissue. If cold water is unavailable, use any cold liquid you have available to reduce the burned skin's temperature.

 CAUTION: DO NOT

- cool more than 20 percent of an adult's body surface area (10 percent for a child) except to extinguish flames.

2. Relieve pain and inflammation with aspirin or ibuprofen. Acetaminophen relieves pain but not inflammation. Keep a burned extremity elevated to reduce gravity-induced swelling.
3. Apply a thin layer of ointment such as bacitracin. Topical antibiotic therapy like bacitracin does not sterilize a wound, but it does decrease the number of bacteria to a level that can be controlled by the body's defense mechanisms and prevents the entrance of bacteria.

 CAUTION: DO NOT

- break any blisters. Intact blisters serve as excellent burn dressings. Cover a ruptured blister with bacitracin ointment and a dry, sterile dressing.
- apply salve, ointment, grease, butter, cream, spray, home remedy, or any other coating on a burn until it has cooled. Such coatings are unsterile and may lead to infection. They can also seal in heat, causing further damage. For moderate and severe burns, a physician will have to scrape off the coating, which will cause the victim unnecessary additional pain.
- place a moist dressing over a burn since it will dry out quickly. A wet dressing over a large area can induce hypothermia. A cold wet pack can be used to cool a burn initially, but it should not serve as a dressing.

- use plastic as a dressing (its only advantage is that it will not stick to the burn), since it will trap moisture and provide a good place for bacteria to grow.

4. Cover the burn with a dry, nonsticking, sterile dressing or a clean cloth. Covering the burn reduces the amount of pain by keeping air from the exposed nerve endings. The main purpose of a dressing over a burn is to keep the burn clean, prevent evaporative loss, and reduce the pain.

Care of Third-Degree Burns

It usually is not necessary to apply cold to third-degree burns since pain is absent. Any pain felt with a third-degree burn comes from accompanying first- and second-degree burns, for which cold applications can be helpful.

1. Cover the burn with a dry, nonsticking, sterile dressing or a clean cloth.

 CAUTION: DO NOT

- apply salve, ointment, grease, butter, cream, spray, home remedy, or any other coating on a burn. Such coatings are unsterile and may lead to infection. They can also seal in the heat, causing further damage. For moderate and severe burns, a physician will have to scrape off the coating, which will cause the victim unnecessary additional pain.

2. Treat the victim for shock by elevating the legs and keeping the victim warm with a clean sheet or blanket.

Chemical Burns

A chemical burn is the result of a caustic or corrosive substance touching the skin. Since chemicals continue to "burn" as long as they are in contact with the skin, they should be removed from the victim as rapidly as possible.

THERMAL BURNS

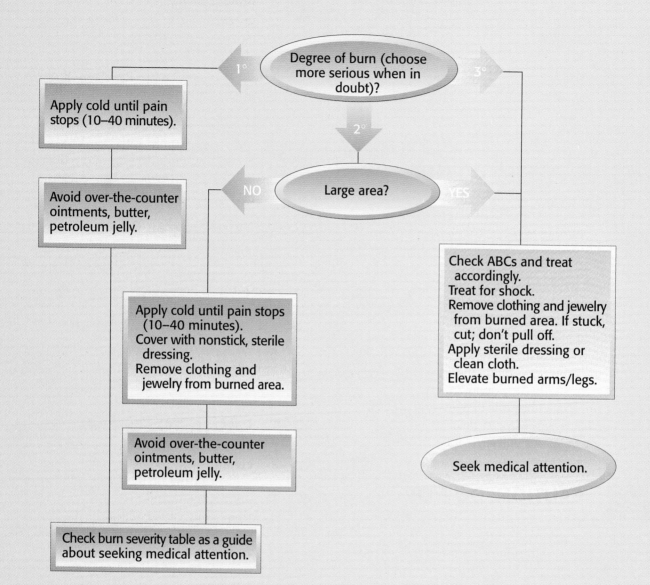

Degree of burn (choose more serious when in doubt)?

1°

Apply cold until pain stops (10–40 minutes).

Avoid over-the-counter ointments, butter, petroleum jelly.

2°

Large area?

NO

Apply cold until pain stops (10–40 minutes).
Cover with nonstick, sterile dressing.
Remove clothing and jewelry from burned area.

Avoid over-the-counter ointments, butter, petroleum jelly.

Check burn severity table as a guide about seeking medical attention.

3° / **YES**

Check ABCs and treat accordingly.
Treat for shock.
Remove clothing and jewelry from burned area. If stuck, cut; don't pull off.
Apply sterile dressing or clean cloth.
Elevate burned arms/legs.

Seek medical attention.

First aid is the same for all chemical burns, except a few specific ones for which a chemical neutralizer has to be used. Alkalies (e.g., drain cleaners) cause more serious burns than acids (e.g., battery acid) because they penetrate deeper and remain active longer. Organic compounds (e.g., petroleum products) are also capable of burning.

What to Do

1. Immediately remove the chemical by flushing with water. If available, use a hose or a shower. Brush dry powder chemicals from the skin *before* flushing, unless large amounts of water are immediately available. Water may activate a dry chemical and cause more damage to the skin. Take precautions to protect yourself from exposure to the chemical.
2. Remove the victim's contaminated clothing while flushing with water. Clothing can hold chemicals, allowing them to continue to burn as long as they are in contact with the skin.
3. Flush for 20 minutes or longer. Let the victim wash with a mild soap before a final rinse. Dilution with large amounts of water decreases the chemical concentration and washes it away.

CAUTION: DO NOT

- waste time! A chemical burn is an emergency!
- apply water under high pressure—it will drive the chemical deeper into the tissue.
- try to neutralize a chemical even if you know which chemical is involved— heat may be produced, resulting in more damage. Some product labels for neutralizing may be wrong. Save the container or the label for the chemical's name.

4. Cover the burned area with a dry, sterile dressing or, for large areas, a clean pillowcase.
5. If the chemical is in an eye, flood it for at least 20 minutes, using low pressure.
6. Seek medical attention immediately for all chemical burns.

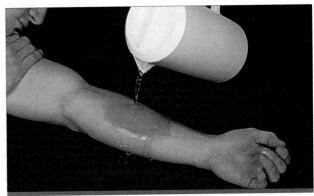

Flooding a chemical burn

Electrocution

Even a mild electrical shock can cause serious internal injuries. A current of 1,000 volts or more is considered high voltage, but even the 110 volts found in ordinary household current can be deadly.

There are three types of electrical injuries: thermal (flame), arc (flash), and true electrical injury (contact). A *thermal burn* (flame) results when clothing or objects in direct contact with the skin are ignited by an electrical current. These injuries are caused by the flames produced by the electrical current and not by the passage of the electrical current or arc.

An *arc burn* (flash) occurs from electricity jumping, or arcing, from one spot to another and

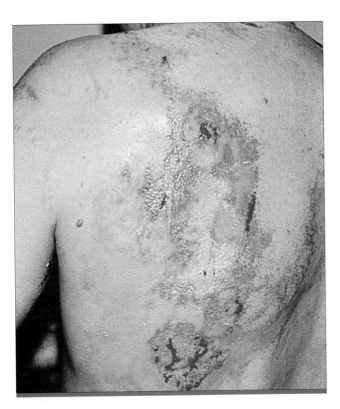

Chemical burn from sulfuric acid

CHEMICAL BURNS

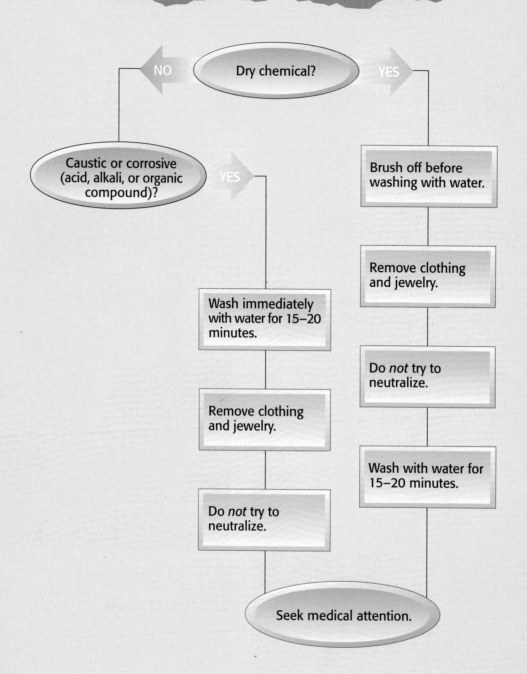

Dry chemical?

NO ← → **YES**

Caustic or corrosive (acid, alkali, or organic compound)? **YES** →

Brush off before washing with water.

Remove clothing and jewelry.

Do *not* try to neutralize.

Wash with water for 15–20 minutes.

Wash immediately with water for 15–20 minutes.

Remove clothing and jewelry.

Do *not* try to neutralize.

Seek medical attention.

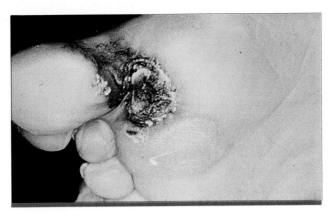

Electrical burn on toe

not from the passage of an electrical current through the body. Although the duration of the flash may be brief, it usually causes extensive superficial injuries.

A *true electrical injury* (contact) happens when an electric current has truly passed through the body. This type of injury is characterized by an entrance wound and an exit wound. The important factor with this type of injury is that the surface injury may be just the tip of the iceberg. High-voltage electrical currents passing through the body may

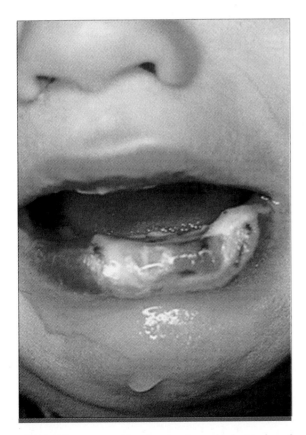

Electrical burn caused by chewing through electrical cord

disrupt the normal heart rhythm and cause cardiac arrest, burns, and other injuries.

During an electric shock, electricity enters the body at the point of contact and travels along the path of least resistance (nerves and blood vessels). The major damage occurs inside the body—the outside burn may appear small. Usually, the electricity exits where the body is touching a surface or is in contact with a ground (e.g., a metal object). Sometimes, a victim has more than one exit site.

What to Do

1. Make sure the area is safe. Unplug, disconnect, or turn off the power. If that is impossible, call the power company or the EMS for help.
2. Check the ABCDs.
3. If the victim fell, check for a spine injury.
4. Treat the victim for shock by elevating the legs 8–12 inches and prevent heat loss by covering the victim with a coat or blanket.
5. Seek medical attention immediately. The ABA recommends that electrical injuries be treated in a burn center.

Contact with a Power Line (Outdoors)

If the electric shock is from contact with a downed power line, the power *must* be turned off before a rescuer approaches anyone who may be in contact with the wire.

If as you approach a victim you feel a tingling sensation in your legs and lower body, stop. The sensation signals that you are on energized ground and that an electrical current is entering through one foot, passing through your lower body, and leaving through the other foot. Raise one foot off the ground, turn around, and hop to a safe place.

If you can safely reach the victim, do not attempt to move any wires, even with wooden poles, tools with wood handles, or tree branches. Do not use objects with a high moisture content and certainly not metal objects. The recommendation for not using wood-handled rakes, brooms, or shovels is that if the voltage is high enough (you seldom will know how much voltage is involved) those objects can conduct electricity and the rescuer will be electrocuted. Do not attempt to move downed wires at all unless you are trained and are equipped with tools able to handle the high voltage.

Wait until trained personnel with the proper equipment can cut the wires or disconnect them. Prevent bystanders from entering the danger area.

ELECTROCUTION

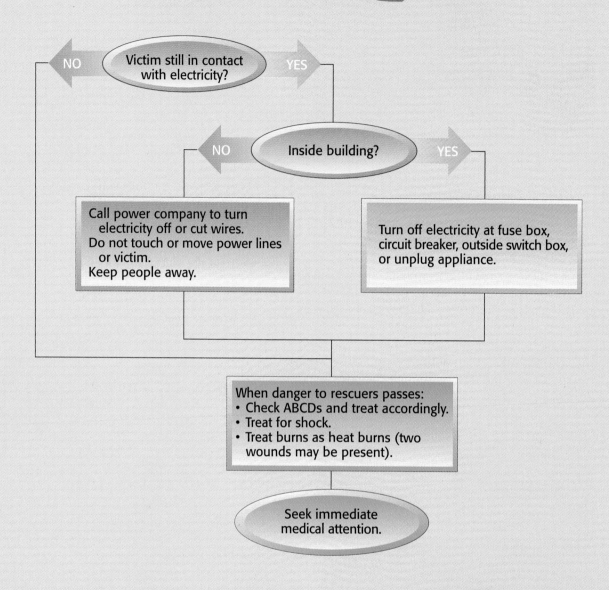

Victim still in contact with electricity?

NO ◄ ► **YES**

Inside building?

NO ◄ ► **YES**

Call power company to turn electricity off or cut wires.
Do not touch or move power lines or victim.
Keep people away.

Turn off electricity at fuse box, circuit breaker, outside switch box, or unplug appliance.

When danger to rescuers passes:
• Check ABCDs and treat accordingly.
• Treat for shock.
• Treat burns as heat burns (two wounds may be present).

Seek immediate medical attention.

Contact inside Buildings

Most electrical burns that occur indoors are caused by faulty electrical equipment or careless use of electrical appliances. Turn off the electricity at the circuit breaker, fuse box, or outside switch box or unplug the appliance if the plug is undamaged. Do not touch the appliance or the victim until the current is off.

Once there is no danger to rescuers, first aid can begin.

What to Do

1. Check the ABCDs and treat accordingly.
2. Check the victim for burns and treat for shock by elevating the legs 8–12 inches and keeping the victim warm. Most electrical burns are third-degree burns, so cover them with a sterile dressing and elevate the affected part.

Electrical current flows quickly into the body's tissues, then exits. The surface injuries of the skin involve small surface areas (entrance and exit points); the major damage occurs deep under the skin. First aiders must keep that in mind when they treat anyone for electrical shock. All victims of electrical shock should receive immediate medical attention.

Thermal (Heat) Burns

Directions: Circle Yes if you agree with the statement, and circle No if you disagree.

Yes   No   1. Relieve pain and tissue damage from a burn by holding the part in a sink filled with running cold water.

Yes   No   2. Pain and inflammation can be relieved with aspirin or ibuprofen in those who can tolerate these over-the-counter medications.

Yes   No   3. Later, a layer of antibiotic ointment or aloe vera gel can be applied on first- and second-degree burns.

Yes   No   4. Butter can be effective on first- and second-degree burns.

Scenario: Tracy is boiling water to make hot chocolate in the office kitchen. She reaches across the stove for a cup. The sleeve of her blouse touches the flame of the gas burner and ignites, sending fire racing up her arm. Her screams bring you and others racing into the kitchen. She has second-degree burns on about 7 percent of her body. What should you do?

_____

_____

Chemical Burns

Yes   No   1. When washing chemicals off the body, flush with water for at least five minutes.

Yes   No   2. When washing chemicals off the body, use high pressure water.

Yes   No   3. Do not try to neutralize a chemical because more damage may result.

Yes   No   4. Brush dry powder chemicals from the skin before flushing unless large amounts of water are immediately available.

Scenario: A 28-year-old man is using a caustic drain cleaner to unclog a bathroom sink. Fifteen minutes after applying the chemical, he runs water into the sink, but the drain remains clogged. Then contrary to the instructions on the drain cleaner package, he attempts to use a plunger to clear the drain, and the solution in the sink splashes on his arm. What should you do?

_____

_____

Electrocution

Yes   No   1. If a victim is in contact with an outdoor electrical wire, try to move it with a wooden pole or handle.

Yes   No   2. For a victim inside a building, turn off the electricity at the fuse box, circuit-breaker, outside switch box, or unplug the appliance.

Scenario: Steve is trimming hedges using an old electric hedge trimmer, which is falling apart, but works. Because the three-pronged grounding plug is a little wobbly, Steve has connected it to a two-pronged adapter, plugged the adapter into an outlet, and started to work on hedges growing along a metal chain-link fence. Things are going well until Steve reaches for the fence for support, and a powerful electric current shoots through his body, causing him to fall over. When you arrive, he is unresponsive. What do you do?

_____

_____

C H A P T E R 9

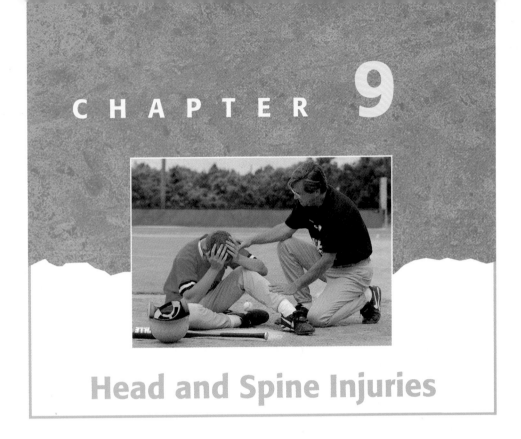

Head and Spine Injuries

Head Injuries

Scalp Wounds

A bleeding scalp wound does not mean the blood supply to the brain is affected. The brain obtains its blood supply from arteries in the neck, not the scalp. Look into the wound for exposed skull bone or brain tissue and indentation of the skull. Suspect a spine injury in the neck area.

What to Do

1. Control bleeding by gently applying direct pressure with a dry sterile dressing. If the dressing becomes blood-filled, do not remove it. Add another dressing on top of the first one.
2. If you suspect a skull fracture, apply pressure around the edges of the wound and over a broad area rather than on the center of the wound. A doughnut (ring) pad serves well in such an application.
3. Keep the head and shoulders slightly elevated to help control bleeding.

 CAUTION: DO NOT

- remove an embedded object; instead stabilize it in place with bulky dressings. If a skull fracture is suspected, do not clean a scalp wound or irrigate it since the fluid can carry debris and bacteria into the brain.

Skull Fracture
What to Look For

It is extremely difficult to determine a skull fracture except by x-ray unless the skull deformity is severe and obvious. Signs of a skull fracture include the following:

- Pain at the point of injury
- Deformity of the skull
- Bleeding from the ears or nose
- Leakage of clear, pink, watery fluid—cerebrospinal fluid (CSF)—from an ear or the nose. To determine if CSF is leaking, have the suspected fluid drip onto a handkerchief, pillowcase, or other cloth. CSF will form a pink ring resembling a target around a slightly blood-tinged center; this is called the "halo sign" or "ring sign"
- Discoloration around the eyes ("raccoon eyes") appearing several hours after the injury
- Discoloration behind an ear (known as "Battle's sign"), appearing several hours after the injury
- Unequal pupils
- Profuse scalp bleeding if skin is broken. A scalp wound may expose the skull or brain tissue
- Penetrating wound (e.g., from a bullet) or impaled object

....

▼ **CAUTION: DO NOT**

- **stop the flow of blood or CSF from an ear or nose. Blocking the flow could increase pressure within the skull.**
- **remove an impaled object from the head. Stabilize it in place with bulky dressings.**
- **clean an open skull fracture—infection of the brain could result.**

....

What to Do

1. Monitor the ABCDs.
2. Cover wounds with a sterile dressing.
3. Stabilize the victim's neck against movement.

4. Slightly elevate the victim's head and shoulders to help control bleeding.
5. Apply pressure around the edges of the wound, not directly on it.

Brain Injuries

When the head is struck with sufficient force, the brain is bounced around inside the skull.

The brain, like other body tissue, will swell when injured. Unlike other tissue, the brain is confined in the skull where little additional space exists to accommodate any swelling. Therefore, swelling of brain tissue or accumulation of blood inside the skull compresses the brain and increases the pressure inside the skull. That pressure causes changes that interfere with brain functioning.

What to Look For

Assessment is directed at determining whether injured brain tissue is swelling. The following signs and symptoms, which may go unnoticed for the first 6–18 hours after injury, are indicative of increased brain swelling.

- Level of responsiveness V, P, or U on the AVPU scale (see page 15). Loss of responsiveness may be short or may persist for hours or days. The victim may alternate between periods of responsiveness and unresponsiveness or be responsive but disoriented, confused, and incoherent.
- Memory loss
- Vomiting and nausea
- Headache
- Vision disturbance. Victim sees "double," or eyes fail to move together
- Unequal pupils
- Weakness, loss of balance, or paralysis
- Seizures
- Blood or CSF leaking from ears or nose
- Combativeness. The victim strikes out randomly and with surprising strength at the nearest person.

For a responsive victim, ask what day it is, where he or she is, and personal questions such as birthday and home address. If the victim cannot answer those questions, there may be a significant problem.

What to Do

1. Seek immediate medical attention for all brain-injury victims.

2. Suspect a spine injury in an unresponsive victim until proved otherwise. See page 85 on how to stabilize the victim's head and neck.

3. Monitor the ABCDs.

4. Control scalp bleeding by covering wounds with sterile dressings as a barrier against infection. If you suspect a skull fracture, apply pressure around the wound edges, not directly on the wound. Do not try to clean a scalp wound of a suspected skull fracture. Stabilize impaled objects in place. Do not try to stop blood or CSF draining from the ears or nose. Blocking either flow could increase pressure within the skull.

5. Brain-injury victims tend to vomit. Rolling the victim onto his or her side while stabilizing the neck against movement will help drain vomit while keeping the airway open.

6. Keep the victim in a slightly head-elevated position to prevent increased blood pressure. If the victim is unconscious, positioning on the side is best for possible vomiting and to keep the airway open.

7. The victim's level of responsiveness or mental status is one of the best indicators of neurologic function. Observations over the first 24 hours may offer clues to problems. Use the mnemonic AVPU (see page 15) to assess and describe a victim's mental status. It is especially helpful with small children who don't talk.

Unfortunately, there is little a first aider can do for a brain injury. The victim must be transported to the care of a neurosurgeon.

 CAUTION: DO NOT

- stop the flow of blood or CSF from the ears or nose. Blocking either flow could increase pressure inside the skull.
- elevate the legs—that might increase pressure in the skull.
- clean an open skull injury—infection of the brain may result.

Head Injury Follow-Up

If any of the following signs appear within 48 hours of a head injury, seek medical attention:

- *Headache.* Expect a headache. If it lasts more than one or two days or increases in severity, however, seek medical advice.

- *Nausea, vomiting.* If nausea lasts more than two hours, seek medical advice. Vomiting once or twice, especially in children, may be expected after a head injury. Vomiting does not tell anything about the severity of the injury. However, if vomiting begins again hours after one or two episodes have ceased, consult a physician.

- *Drowsiness.* Allow a victim to sleep, but wake the victim at least every two hours to check the state of consciousness and sense of orientation by asking his or her name, address, telephone number, and an information-processing question (e.g., adding or multiplying numbers). If the victim cannot answer correctly or appears confused or disoriented, call a physician.

- *Vision problems.* If the victim "sees double," if the eyes fail to move together, or if one pupil appears to be larger than the other, seek medical advice.

- *Mobility.* If the victim cannot use his or her arms or legs as well as previously or is unsteady in walking, medical care should be sought.

- *Speech.* If the victim has slurred speech or is unable to talk, a doctor should be consulted.

- *Seizures or convulsions.* If the victim has a violent involuntary contraction (spasm) or series of contractions of the skeletal muscles, seek medical assistance.

Eye Injuries

 CAUTION: DO NOT

- assume that any eye injury is innocent. When in doubt, seek medical attention immediately.

Penetrating Injuries

Penetrating eye injuries are relatively common, severe injuries that result when a sharp object, such as a knife or a needle, penetrates the eye and then is withdrawn or when pieces from a tool enter the eye and lodge there as foreign bodies.

What to Do

1. Seek immediate medical attention. Any penetrating eye injury should be managed in the hospital.

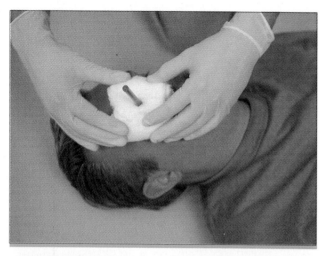

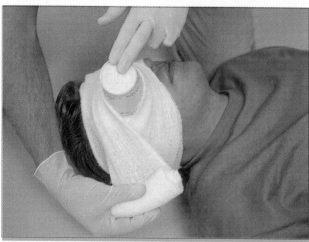

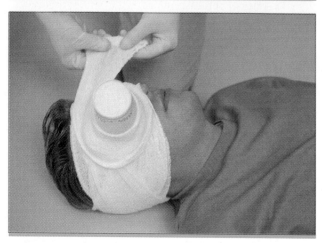

Protecting a long penetrating object against movement (using paper cup)

CAUTION: DO NOT

- remove an object stuck in the eye or try to wash out an object with water.
- exert pressure on an injured eyeball or a penetrating object.

2. Protect the injured eye with a paper cup, cardboard folded into a cone, or a doughnut-shaped pad made from a roller gauze bandage or a cravat bandage to prevent the object from being driven deeper into the eye.
3. Cover the undamaged eye to stop movement of the damaged eye (known as sympathetic eye movement).

Blows to the Eye

Blunt trauma varies in severity from negligible to sight threatening.

What to Do

1. Apply an ice pack immediately for about 15 minutes to reduce pain and swelling. Do not exert any pressure on the eye.
2. Seek medical attention immediately in cases of pain, reduced vision, or discoloration (a black eye).

Cuts of the Eye and Lid

What to Do

1. Bandage both eyes lightly.
2. Seek medical attention immediately.

Chemical Burns

Chemical burns of the eyes are extremely sight threatening. In such cases, first aid can determine the fate of the eye and vision.

Alkalies cause greater damage than acids because they penetrate deeper and continue to burn longer. Common alkalies include drain cleaners, cleaning agents, ammonia, cement, plaster, and caustic soda. Common acids include hydrochloric acid, nitric acid, sulfuric (battery) acid, and acetic acid.

Damage can happen in one to five minutes, so speed in removing the chemical is vital.

What to Do

1. Use your fingers to keep the eye open as wide as possible.
2. Flush the eye with water immediately. If possible, use warm water. If water is not available, use any nonirritating liquid.

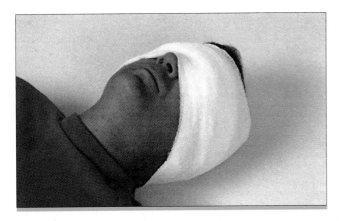

Bandaging both eyes stops sympathetic eye movement.

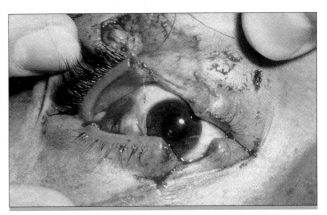

Lacerated eyelid

What to Do

1. Cover the eye loosely with a sterile dressing that has been moistened with clean water. Do *not* try to push the eyeball back into the socket.
2. Protect the injured eye with a paper cup, cardboard folded into a cone, or a doughnut-shaped pad made from a roller gauze bandage or a cravat bandage.
3. Cover the undamaged eye with a patch to stop movement of the damaged eye (known as sympathetic eye movement).
4. Seek medical attention immediately.

Foreign Objects

Try one or more of the following, starting with number 1.

What to Do

1. Lift the upper lid over the lower lid, allowing the lashes to brush the object off the inside of the upper lid. Have the victim blink a few times and let the eye move the object out. If the object remains, keep the eye closed.

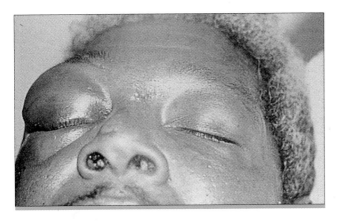

Blow to the eye

- Hold the victim's head under a faucet or pour water into the eye from any clean container for at least 20 minutes, continuously and gently. You cannot use too much water on these injuries.
- Irrigate from the nose side of the eye toward the outside, to avoid flushing material into the other eye.
- Tell the victim to roll the eyeball as much as possible to help wash out the eye.

3. Loosely bandage both eyes with cold, wet dressings.
4. Seek immediate medical attention.

 CAUTION: DO NOT
- **try to neutralize the chemical. Water usually is readily available and better for eye irrigation.**
- **use an eye cup for a chemical burn.**

Eye Knocked Out

A blow to the eye can avulse it (knock it out) from its socket.

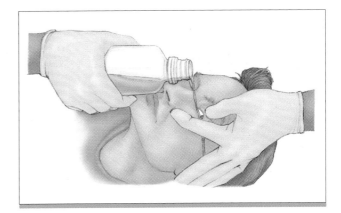

Flushing eye for chemical burn

2. Try flushing the object out by rinsing the eye gently with warm water. Hold the eyelid open and tell the victim to move the eye as it is rinsed.

3. Examine the lower lid by pulling it down gently. If you can see the object, remove it with a moistened sterile gauze or clean cloth.

4. Many foreign bodies lodge under the upper eyelid, requiring some expertise in everting the lid and removing the object. Examine the upper lid by grasping the lashes of the upper lid, placing a match stick or cotton-tipped swab across the upper lid and roll the lid upward over the stick or swab. If you can see the object, remove it with a moistened sterile gauze or clean cloth.

CAUTION: DO NOT

- allow the victim to rub the eye.
- try to remove an embedded foreign object.
- use dry cotton (cotton balls or cotton-tipped swabs) or instruments (e.g., tweezers) on an eye.

Eye Burns from Light
Burns can result if a person looks at a source of ultraviolet light (e.g., sunlight, arc welding, bright snow, tanning lamps). Severe pain happens one to six hours after exposure.

1. Cover both eyes with cold, wet packs. Tell the victim not to rub the eyes.

2. Have the victim rest in a darkened room. Do not allow light to reach the victim's eyes.

3. Give an aspirin, acetaminophen, or ibuprofen for pain, if needed.

4. Call an ophthalmologist for advice.

Nose Injuries
Nosebleeds
There are two types of nosebleeds:

- *Anterior (front of nose)* is the most common type (90 percent). Blood comes out of the nose through one nostril.
- *Posterior (back of nose)* type involves massive bleeding backward into the mouth or down the back of the throat. A posterior nosebleed is serious and requires medical attention.

CAUTION: DO NOT

- allow the victim to tilt the head backward.
- probe the nose with a cotton-tipped swab.
- move the victim's head and neck if a spine injury is suspected.

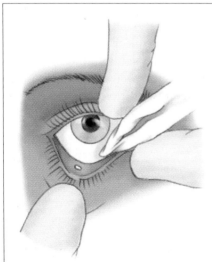

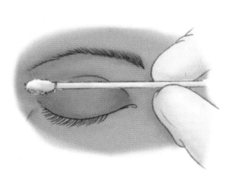

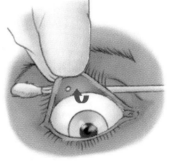

a. If tears or gentle flushing do not remove object, gently pull lower lid down. Remove an object by gently flushing with lukewarm water or a wet sterile gauze.

b. Tell the person to look down. Pull gently downward on upper eyelashes. Lay a swab or match stick across the top of the lid.

c. Fold the lid over the swab or matchstick. Remove an object by gently flushing with lukewarm water or a wet sterile gauze.

Removing foreign object from the eye

EYE INJURIES

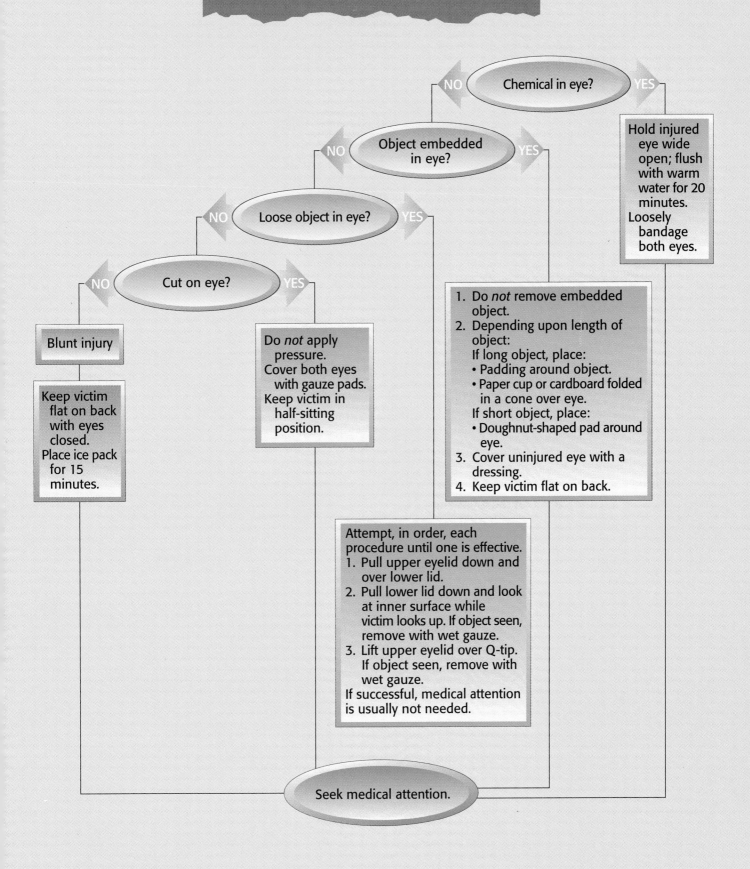

Chemical in eye?
NO / YES

YES: Hold injured eye wide open; flush with warm water for 20 minutes. Loosely bandage both eyes.

Object embedded in eye?
NO / YES

YES:
1. Do *not* remove embedded object.
2. Depending upon length of object:
   If long object, place:
   • Padding around object.
   • Paper cup or cardboard folded in a cone over eye.
   If short object, place:
   • Doughnut-shaped pad around eye.
3. Cover uninjured eye with a dressing.
4. Keep victim flat on back.

Loose object in eye?
NO / YES

YES:
Attempt, in order, each procedure until one is effective.
1. Pull upper eyelid down and over lower lid.
2. Pull lower lid down and look at inner surface while victim looks up. If object seen, remove with wet gauze.
3. Lift upper eyelid over Q-tip. If object seen, remove with wet gauze.
If successful, medical attention is usually not needed.

Cut on eye?
NO / YES

YES:
Do *not* apply pressure.
Cover both eyes with gauze pads.
Keep victim in half-sitting position.

NO: Blunt injury
Keep victim flat on back with eyes closed.
Place ice pack for 15 minutes.

Seek medical attention.

What to Do

1. Keep the victim in a sitting-up position to reduce blood pressure.
2. Keep the victim's head tilted slightly forward so blood can run out the front of the nose, not down the back of the throat, which can cause choking, nausea, or vomiting. Vomit could be inhaled into the lungs.
3. Pinch (or have the victim pinch) both nostrils with steady pressure for five minutes. Remind the victim to breathe through the mouth and to spit out any accumulated blood.
4. If bleeding persists, have the victim gently blow the nose to remove any irregular clots and excess blood and to minimize sneezing. This allows new clots to form. Then pinch the nostrils again for five minutes.
5. You might try one of the following methods in conjunction with nose pinching:
   • Place a roll of gauze (the diameter of a pencil) between the upper lip and the teeth. Press against the gauze roll with your fingers to stop the blood flow.
   • Apply an ice pack over the nose area to help control bleeding—especially if caused by a blow to the nose.
6. Place an unconscious victim on his or her side to prevent inhaling of blood and try the procedures listed above.
7. Seek medical attention if any of the following applies:
   • The nostril pinching and other methods do not stop the bleeding.
   • You suspect a posterior nosebleed.
   • The victim has high blood pressure or is taking anticoagulants (blood thinners) or large doses of aspirin.
   • Bleeding happens after a blow to the nose, and you suspect a broken nose.

Broken Nose

1. Seek medical attention.
2. Treat a nosebleed as described above.
3. Apply an ice pack to the nose for 15 minutes. Do not try to straighten a crooked nose.

Dental Injuries

Because dental emergencies generally cause considerable pain and anxiety, managing them promptly can provide great relief to the victim.

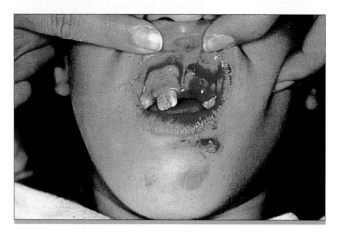
Tooth knocked out

Knocked-Out Tooth

1. Have the victim rinse his or her mouth and put a rolled gauze pad in the socket to control bleeding.
2. Find the tooth and handle it by the crown, never the root, to minimize damage to the ligament fibers.
3. The best place for a knocked-out tooth is its socket. A tooth often can be successfully reimplanted if it has been put back in its socket within 30 minutes after the injury.

   Try to replace the tooth into the socket, using adjacent teeth as a guide. Push down on the tooth so the top is even with the adjacent teeth. Biting down gently on gauze is helpful.

 CAUTION: DO NOT

• handle a knocked-out tooth roughly.
• put a knocked-out tooth in water, mouthwash, alcohol, or Betadine.
• put a knocked-out tooth in skim milk, reconstituted powdered milk, or milk by-products such as yogurt.
• rinse a knocked-out tooth unless you are reinserting it in the socket.
• place a knocked-out tooth in anything that can dry or crush the outside of the tooth.
• scrub a knocked-out tooth or remove any attached tissue fragments.
• remove a partially extracted tooth. Push it back into place and seek a dentist so the loose tooth can be stabilized.

DENTAL INJURIES

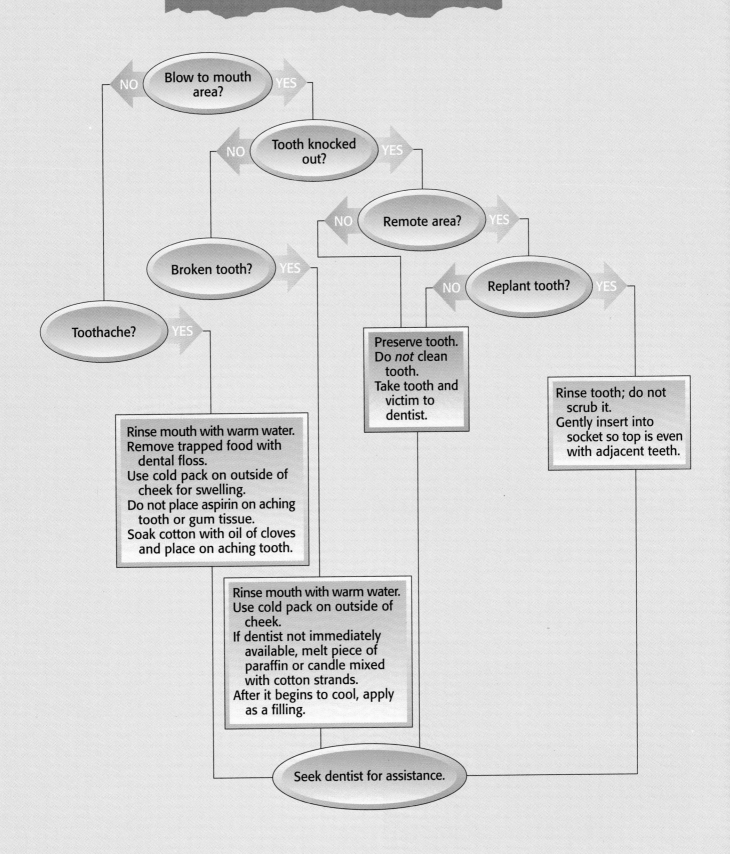

Blow to mouth area? NO / YES

Tooth knocked out? NO / YES

Remote area? NO / YES

Broken tooth? YES

Replant tooth? NO / YES

Toothache? YES

Preserve tooth.
Do *not* clean tooth.
Take tooth and victim to dentist.

Rinse tooth; do not scrub it.
Gently insert into socket so top is even with adjacent teeth.

Rinse mouth with warm water.
Remove trapped food with dental floss.
Use cold pack on outside of cheek for swelling.
Do not place aspirin on aching tooth or gum tissue.
Soak cotton with oil of cloves and place on aching tooth.

Rinse mouth with warm water.
Use cold pack on outside of cheek.
If dentist not immediately available, melt piece of paraffin or candle mixed with cotton strands.
After it begins to cool, apply as a filling.

Seek dentist for assistance.

When immediate reinsertion is not possible, one of the worst things you can do to a knocked-out tooth is to transport it dry. Consider using saliva for the short term (less than one hour).

The best transport medium is Save-a-Tooth™ kit. Its use extends the viability of the ligament fibers for 6 to 12 hours.

Some experts recommend that the tooth be placed in the victim's mouth to keep it moist until dental treatment is available. This method, though convenient, presents the risk, especially in children, of the tooth's being accidentally swallowed.

4. Take the victim and the tooth to a dentist immediately.

Broken Tooth

What to Do

1. Gently clean dirt and blood from the injured area with a sterile gauze pad or a clean cloth and warm water.

2. If you are in a remote area with no dentist nearby, you can make a temporary cap from melted candle wax or paraffin and a few strands of cotton. When the wax begins to harden but can still be molded, press a wad of it onto the tooth. Other improvisations include using ski wax or chewing gum (preferably sugarless).

3. Apply an ice pack on the face in the area of the injured tooth, to decrease swelling.

4. If you suspect a jaw fracture, stabilize the jaw by tying a bandage wrapped under the chin and over the top of the head.

5. Seek a dentist immediately.

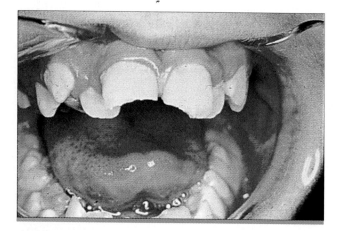

Broken teeth

Toothache

The tooth will be sensitive to heat and cold. Identify the diseased tooth by tapping the area with a spoon handle or similar object. A diseased tooth will hurt.

What to Do

1. Rinse the mouth with warm water to clean it out.

2. Use dental floss to remove any food that might be trapped between the teeth.

3. If you suspect a cavity, insert a small cotton ball soaked in oil of cloves (eugenol) to help depress the pain. Take care to keep the oil off the gums, lips, and inside surfaces of the cheeks. If applicable, follow the same procedures as for a broken tooth.

4. Give the victim an analgesic (aspirin, acetaminophen, or ibuprofen) to reduce pain.

5. Seek a dentist immediately.

 CAUTION: DO NOT

- place aspirin, acetaminophen, or ibuprofen on the aching tooth or gum tissues or allow them to dissolve in the mouth. A serious acid burn can result.

- cover a cavity with cotton if there is any pus discharge or facial swelling. See a dentist immediately.

- stick anything into the exposed cavity or into the softened exposed root.

Spine Injuries

What to Look For

Head injuries serve as a clue since the head may have been snapped suddenly in one or more directions, endangering the spine.

- Painful movement of the arms or legs
- Numbness, tingling, weakness, or burning sensation in the arms or legs
- Loss of bowel or bladder control
- Paralysis of the arms or legs
- Deformity (odd-looking angle of the victim's head and neck)
- Use the Skill Scan: Checking for Spine Injuries on page 83

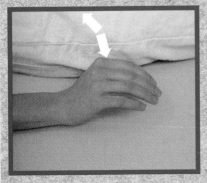

1.

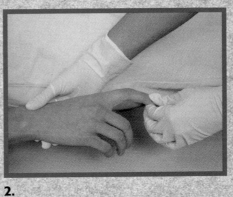

2.

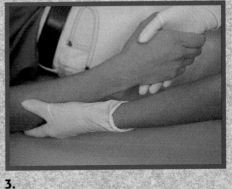

3.

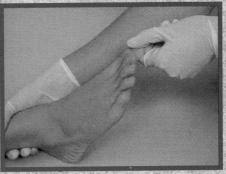

4.

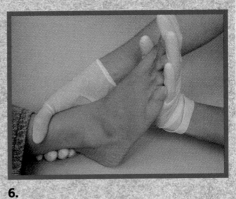

5.

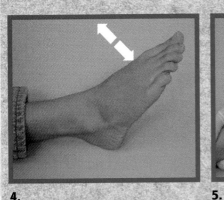

6.

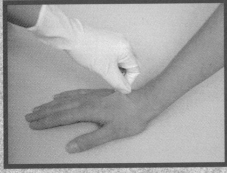

7.

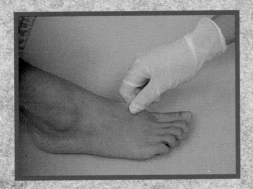

8.

Conscious Victim—
Upper Extremity Checks
1. Victim wiggles fingers.
2. Rescuer touches fingers.
3. Victim squeezes rescuer's hand.

Conscious Victim—
Lower-Extremity Checks
4. Victim wiggles toes.
5. Rescuer touches toes.
6. Victim pushes foot against rescuer's hand.

Victim's failure to perform may mean spine injury!

Unconscious Victim
7. Pinch hand.
8. Pinch foot.

Ask a responsive victim these questions:

- *Is there pain?* Neck (cervical spine) injuries radiate pain to the arms; upper-back (thoracic spine) injuries radiate pain around the ribs; lower-back injuries usually radiate pain down the legs. Often, the victim will describe the pain as "electric."

- *Can you move your feet?* Ask the victim to press a foot against your hand. If the victim cannot perform this movement or if the movement is extremely weak against your hand, the victim may have injured the spine.

- *Can you move your fingers?* Moving the fingers is a sign that nerve pathways are intact. Ask the victim to grip your hand. A strong grip indicates that a spine injury is unlikely.

If the victim is unresponsive, do the following:

- Look for cuts, bruises, and deformities.

- Test responses by pinching the victim's hand (either palm or back of the hand) and bare foot (sole or top of the foot). No reaction could mean spine damage.

- Ask bystanders what happened. If you still are not sure about a possible spine injury, assume the victim has one until it is proved otherwise.

What to Do

1. Check and monitor the ABCDs. For an unresponsive victim, use the procedures described on page 25 for opening the airway.

2. Stabilize the victim against any movement, using one of the following methods. Whatever method you use, tell the victim not to move.
   - Grasp the victim's clavicle and trapezius muscle (shoulder) and cradle the head between the inside of your forearms. Hold the victim's head and neck still until the EMS responds.
   - Grasp the victim's head over the ears and hold the head and neck still until the EMS responds.
   - If a long wait for the EMS to respond is anticipated or if you are tired from holding the victim's head in place, kneel with the victim's head between your knees or place objects on each side of the victim's head to prevent it from rolling from side to side.

 CAUTION: DO NOT

- move the victim, even if the victim is in water. Wait for the EMS to arrive—they have the proper training and equipment. Victims with suspected spine injury require cervical collars and stabilization on a spine board. It is better to do nothing than to mishandle a victim with a spine injury.

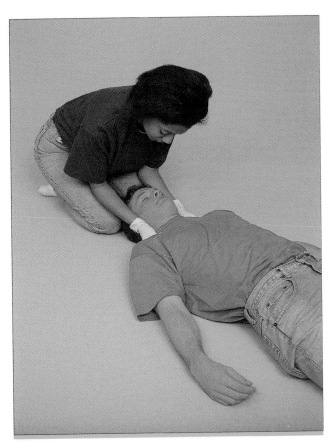

Stabilize against movement by holding onto shoulders and gently squeeze head between arms.

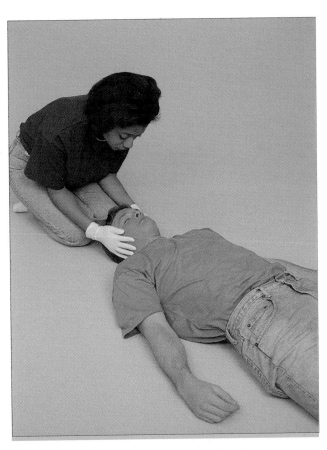

Stabilize against movement by holding the head.

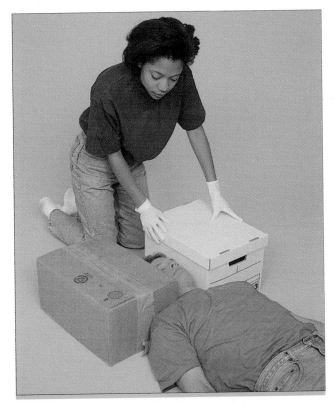

Stabilize against movement by placing objects on each side of the head.

Head Injuries

Directions: Circle Yes if you agree with the statement, and circle No if you disagree.

Yes No   1. For a suspected skull fracture, press around the edges and not directly on the wound.

Yes No   2. Do NOT remove impaled (embedded) objects.

Yes No   3. Head injured victims should be checked for a possible spine injury.

Scenario: At work, you are called to help a carpenter who fell from a ladder. A bystander says that, though responsive now, the victim was previously motionless for a couple of minutes. The victim complains about a severe headache and dizziness. There is swelling on the back of his head. What should you do?

_____

_____

Eye Injuries

Yes No   1. After a blow to an eye, apply a cold pack for about 15 minutes.

Yes No   2. Tears are sufficient to flush a chemical from the eye.

Yes No   3. Use a clean, damp cloth to remove an object off the eyeball's surface.

Scenario: As Sam is attempting to jump-start the company car, a spark from the jump-cables ignites hydrogen gas that has accumulated in the battery. This causes the battery to explode. The battery cap flys off, and battery acid splashes into Sam's eyes. What should you do?

_____

_____

Dental Injuries

Yes No   1. Preserve a knocked-out tooth in mouthwash or rubbing alcohol.

Yes No   2. Scrub a knocked-out tooth before taking the victim to a dentist.

Yes No   3. Sometimes a knocked-out tooth should be reinserted by a first aider.

Scenario: Mike, age 20, was struck in the mouth by a pipe loosely suspended from a cable. He has spit out two of his front teeth, which are lying on the ground. What should you do?

_____

_____

Spine Injuries

Yes No   1. Do NOT move and stabilize against movement a victim with a suspected spine injury.

Yes No   2. Inability of fingers and/or feet to move may indicate a spine injury.

Yes No   3. A head injury may be a reason to suspect a spine injury.

Scenario: You hear a loud crash after a car hit a concrete median. You have made a scene survey. The driver complains of numbness and loss of feeling in both legs. What should you do?

_____

_____

CHAPTER 10

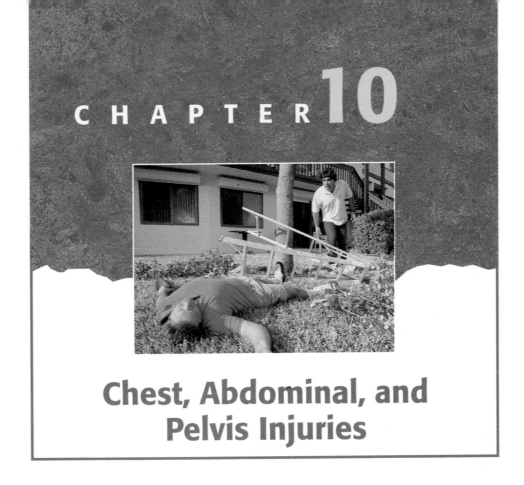

Chest, Abdominal, and Pelvis Injuries

Chest Injuries

All chest injury victims should have their ABCDs checked and rechecked. A responsive chest injury victim usually should be sitting up or placed with the injured side down. That position protects the uninjured side from blood inside the chest cavity and allows the good lung to expand.

To prevent pneumonia, encourage or force victims with chest-wall injuries to clear their lungs at least hourly by coughing, despite the pain.

Rib Fractures

The main symptom of a fractured rib is pain when the victim breathes, coughs, or moves.

What to Do

1. Stabilize the ribs by having the victim hold a pillow or other similar soft object against the injured area. Or you can use bandages to hold the pillow in place or tie an arm over the injured area.
2. Tell the victim to take deep breaths and to cough at least once each hour to prevent pneumonia.
3. Seek medical attention.

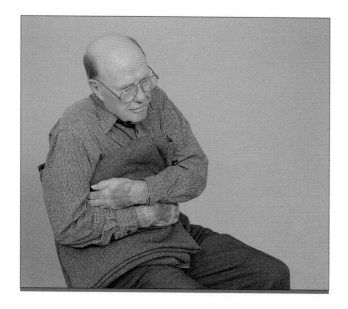

Sucking Chest Wound

A sucking chest wound results when a chest wound allows air to pass into and out of the chest with each breath.

What to Do

1. Have the victim take a breath and let it out; then seal the wound with anything available to stop air from entering the chest cavity. Plastic wrap or a plastic bag works well. Tape it in place with one corner untaped. That creates a flutter valve to prevent air from being trapped in the chest cavity. If plastic wrap is not available, you can use your hand.
2. If the victim has trouble breathing or seems to be getting worse, remove the plastic cover (or your hand) to let air escape, then reapply.
3. Seek medical attention.

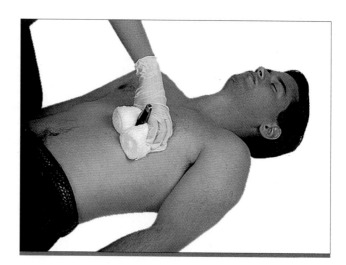

Stabilize penetrating object with bulky padding.

Stabilize chest with soft object such as pillow, coat, or blanket (hold or tie). Tell victim to occasionally take a deep breath and to cough.

Impaled Object in Chest

What to Do

1. Stabilize the object in place with bulky dressings. *Do not try to remove an impaled object*—bleeding and air in the chest cavity can result.
2. Seek medical attention.

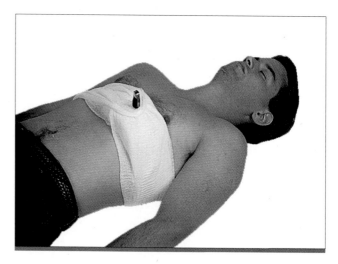

Secure padding and object.

CHEST INJURIES

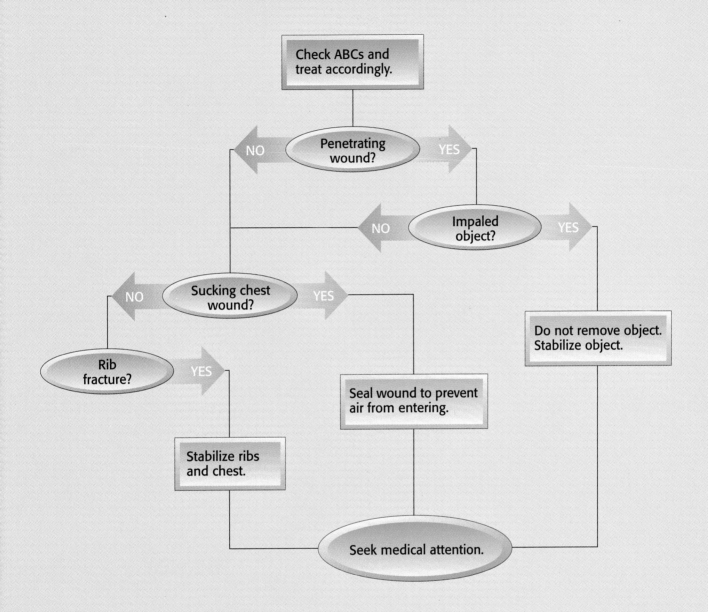

Abdominal Injuries

Blunt Wound

What to Do

1. Place the victim on one side in a comfortable position and expect vomiting. Do not give the victim any food or drink. If you are hours from a medical facility, allow the victim to suck on a clean cloth soaked in water to relieve a dry mouth.
2. Seek medical attention.

Penetrating Wound

Expect internal organs to be damaged.

What to Do

1. If the penetrating object is still in place, stabilize the object and control bleeding by using bulky dressings around it. *Do not try to remove the object.*
2. Seek medical attention.

Protruding Organs

What to Do

1. Cover protruding organs with a sterile dressing or clean cloth.
2. Pour drinkable water on the dressing to keep the organ from drying out.
3. Seek medical attention.

 CAUTION: DO NOT
- try to reinsert protruding organs into the abdomen—you could introduce infection or damage the intestines.
- cover the organs tightly.
- cover the organs with any material that clings or disintegrates when wet.

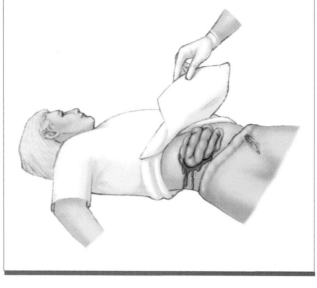

Do not reinsert protruding organs. Cover them with a moist, sterile dressing.

them inward at the iliac crests (upper points of the hips). A fractured pelvis will be painful. See Figures 6a and 6b, on page 17.

What to Do

1. Treat the victim for shock.
2. Place padding between the victim's thighs, then tie the victim's knees and ankles together. If the knees are bent, place padding under them for support.
3. Keep the victim on a firm surface.
4. Seek medical attention.

 CAUTION: DO NOT
- roll the victim—additional internal damage could result.
- move the victim. Whenever possible, wait for the EMS ambulance, with its trained personnel and a backboard.

Pelvis Injuries

To determine if a victim's pelvis is fractured, gently press the sides of the pelvis downward and squeeze

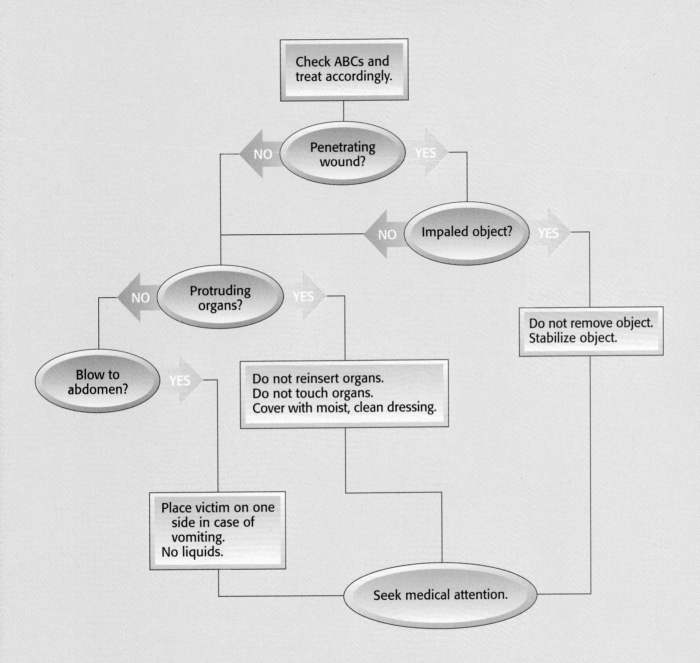

Check ABCs and treat accordingly.

Penetrating wound? — NO / YES

Impaled object? — NO / YES

Protruding organs? — NO / YES

Blow to abdomen? — YES

Do not remove object.
Stabilize object.

Do not reinsert organs.
Do not touch organs.
Cover with moist, clean dressing.

Place victim on one side in case of vomiting.
No liquids.

Seek medical attention.

Chest Injuries

Directions: Circle Yes if you agree with the statement, and circle No if you disagree.

Yes   No   1. Stabilize a rib fracture by strapping (taping) a victim's chest as tight as possible.

Yes   No   2. Stabilize an impaled (embedded) object in the chest with bulking padding to prevent movement.

Yes   No   3. Seal off a chest wound that has air passing in and out of the chest.

Scenario: An iron rod breaks off and sticks into a construction worker's chest while he is tying the rods for a concrete foundation. You are called over to help with the injured worker and you find that the iron rod has been removed. Air is passing into and out of the victim's chest with each breath he takes. What should you do?

_____

_____

_____

Abdominal Injuries

Yes   No   1. Gently push protruding organs back through the abdominal wound.

Yes   No   2. The dressing covering exposed intestines should be kept dry.

Yes   No   3. Remove any penetrating object from the abdomen.

Yes   No   4. For a blow to the abdomen and when internal injuries are suspected, place the victim on his or her side.

Scenario: A 45-year-old repairman falls while carrying a replacement glass for a broken window. The new glass breaks in several jagged pieces. You find him lying on his back with a blood-soaked shirt. You see a lacerated abdomen with several loops of bowel protruding through the laceration. What should you do?

_____

_____

_____

Pelvis Injuries

Yes   No   1. Keep the victim on a firm surface.

Yes   No   2. Keep the victim's knees bent and place padding between the legs.

Scenario: An older secretary slips while on stairs and falls down five steps. She is at the bottom of the stairs lying on her side. You suspect a pelvic fracture because she is complaining about severe pain in the pelvic area. What should you do?

_____

_____

_____

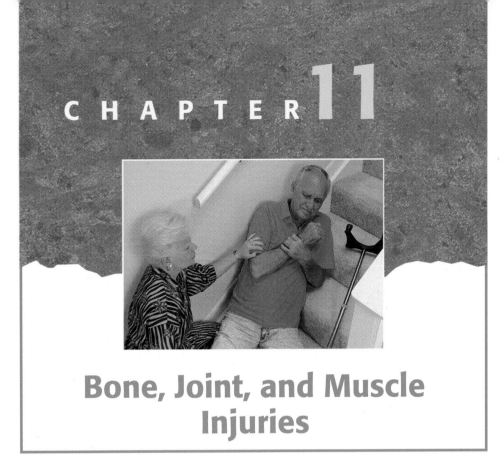

CHAPTER 11

Bone, Joint, and Muscle Injuries

Fractures

The terms fracture and broken bone have the same meaning: a break or crack in a bone. There are two categories of fractures:

- Closed (simple) fracture. The skin is intact and no wound exists anywhere near the fracture site.
- Open (compound) fracture. The overlying skin has been damaged or broken. The wound may be the result of the bone protruding through the skin or of a direct blow that cuts the skin at the time of the fracture. The bone may not always be visible in the wound.

What to Look For

It may be difficult to tell if a bone is fractured. When in doubt, treat the injury as a fracture. Use the mnemonic DOTS (deformity, open wound, tenderness, swelling) found on page 16:

- *Deformity* is not always obvious. Compare the injured part with the uninjured opposite part.
- *Open wound* may indicate an underlying fracture.
- *Tenderness* and pain are commonly found only at the injury site. The victim usually will be able to point to the site of the pain. A useful procedure for detecting a fracture is to gently feel along the bones; victim complaints about pain or tenderness serve as a reliable sign of a fracture.
- *Swelling* caused by bleeding happens rapidly after a fracture.

Additional signs and symptoms include:

- *Loss of use* may or may not occur. "Guarding" occurs when motion produces pain; the victim refuses to use the injured part. Sometimes,

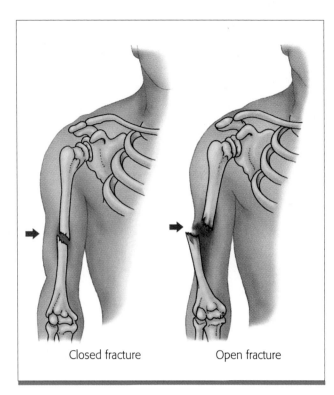

Closed fracture   Open fracture

Fractures

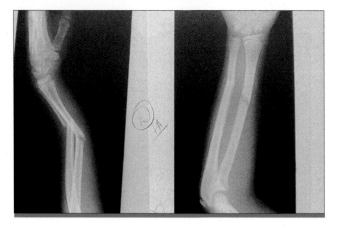

X-rays of victim with forearm fracture before and after setting

however, the victim is able to move a fractured limb with little or no pain.

- A *grating sensation* can be felt and sometimes even heard when the ends of the broken bone rub together. Do *not* move the injured limb in an attempt to detect it.
- *The history of the injury* can lead you to suspect a fracture whenever a serious accident has happened. The victim may have heard or felt the bone snap.

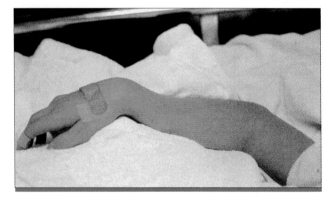

Forearm fracture

What to Do

1. Check and treat ABCDs. Fractures, even open fractures, seldom present an immediate threat to life.
2. Treat the victim for shock.
3. Determine what happened and the location of the injury.
4. Gently remove clothing covering the injured area. Cut clothing at the seams if necessary.
5. Use the mnemonic LAF (look and feel) as a reminder of how to examine an extremity.
   - **L**ook at the injury site. Swelling and black-and-blue marks, which indicate escape of blood into the tissues, may come from either the bone end or associated muscular and blood vessel damage. Shortening or severe deformity (angulation) between the joints or deformity around the joints, shortening of the extremity, and rotation of the extremity when compared with the opposite extremity indicate a bone injury. Lacerations or even small puncture wounds near the site of a bone fracture are considered open fractures.
   - **A**nd
   - **F**eel the injured area. If a fracture is not obvious, gently press, touch, or feel along the length of the bone for deformities, tenderness, and swelling.
6. Check blood flow and nerves. Use the mnemonic CSM (circulation, sensation, movement) as a way of remembering what to do. See page 96.
   - *Circulation.* Feel for the radial pulse (located on the thumb side of the wrist) for an arm injury and the posterior tibial pulse (located be-

tween the inside ankle bone and the Achilles tendon) for a leg injury. A pulseless arm or leg is a significant emergency that requires immediate surgical care.

- *Sensation.* Lightly touch or squeeze the victim's toes or fingers and ask the victim what he or she feels. Loss of sensation is an early sign of nerve damage or spine damage.
- *Movement.* Check for nerve damage by asking the victim to wiggle his or her toes or fingers. If the toes or fingers are injured, do not have the victim attempt to move them.

The major blood vessels of an extremity tend to run close to bone, which means that any time a bone is broken, the adjacent blood vessels are at risk of being torn by bone fragments or pinched off between the ends of the broken bone. The tissues of the arms and legs cannot survive without a continuing blood supply for more than two or three hours. This requires seeking immediate medical attention.

7. Use the RICE (rest-ice-compression-elevation) procedures (see page 99).
8. Use a splint to stabilize the fracture (see Chapter 12).

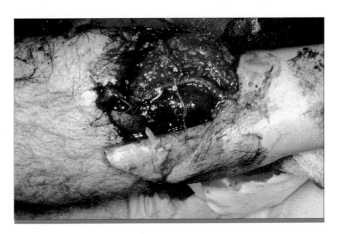

Open tibia, fibula fracture

Joint Injuries
Dislocations

A dislocation occurs when a joint comes apart and stays apart with the bone ends no longer in contact. The shoulders, elbows, fingers, hips, kneecaps, and ankles are the joints most frequently affected. Dislocations have signs and symptoms similar to those of a fracture: deformity, severe pain, swelling, and the inability of the victim to move the injured joint. The main sign of a dislocation is deformity—its ap-

pearance will be different from that of a comparable uninjured joint.

What to Do

1. Check the CSM (circulation, sensation, movement). If the end of the dislocated bone is pressing on nerves or blood vessels, numbness or paralysis may exist below the dislocation. When dealing with a dislocation, always check the pulses. If there is no pulse in the injured extremity, transport the victim to a medical facility immediately.
2. Use the RICE procedures (see page 99).
3. Use a splint to stabilize the joint in the position in which it was found. (See Chapter 12.)
4. Do not try to reduce the joint (put the displaced parts back into their normal positions), since nerve and blood vessel damage could result.
5. Seek medical attention for reduction of the dislocation.

Sprains

A sprain is an injury to a joint in which the ligaments and other tissues are damaged by violent stretching or twisting. Attempts to move or use the joint increase the pain. The skin about the joint may be discolored because of bleeding from torn tissues. It often is difficult to distinguish between a severe sprain and a fracture, because their signs and symptoms are similar.

Treatment consists of rest, ice, compression, and elevation (RICE; see page 99). It is vitally important to keep swelling out of a joint by using cold promptly; it is even more important to make the swelling recede as quickly as possible with a compression (elastic) bandage.

Muscle Injuries
Strains

A muscle strain, also known as a muscle pull, occurs when a muscle is stretched beyond its normal range of motion, resulting in the muscle tearing.

What to Look For

Any of the following signs and symptoms may indicate a muscle strain:

- sharp pain
- extreme tenderness when the area is touched

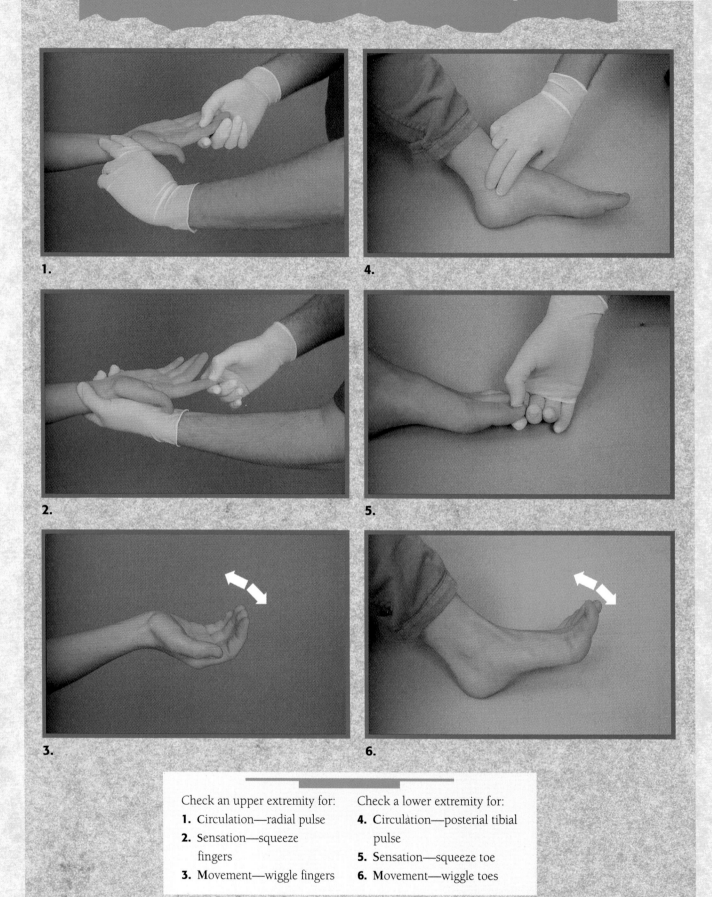

1.

4.

2.

5.

3.

6.

Check an upper extremity for:
1. Circulation—radial pulse
2. Sensation—squeeze fingers
3. Movement—wiggle fingers

Check a lower extremity for:
4. Circulation—posterial tibial pulse
5. Sensation—squeeze toe
6. Movement—wiggle toes

FRACTURES

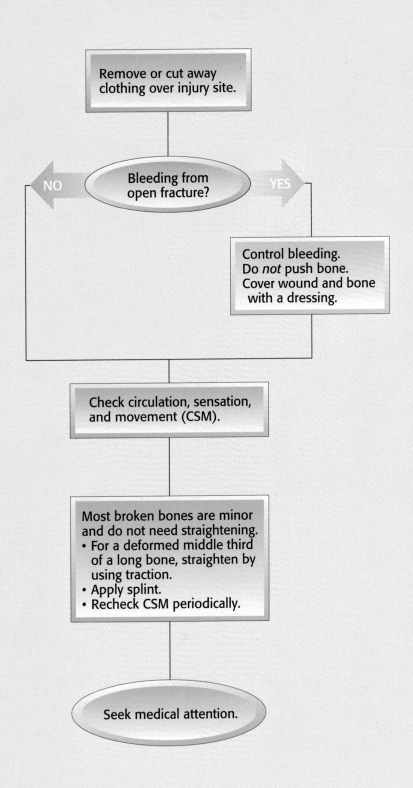

Remove or cut away clothing over injury site.

Bleeding from open fracture?

NO / **YES**

Control bleeding.
Do *not* push bone.
Cover wound and bone with a dressing.

Check circulation, sensation, and movement (CSM).

Most broken bones are minor and do not need straightening.
• For a deformed middle third of a long bone, straighten by using traction.
• Apply splint.
• Recheck CSM periodically.

Seek medical attention.

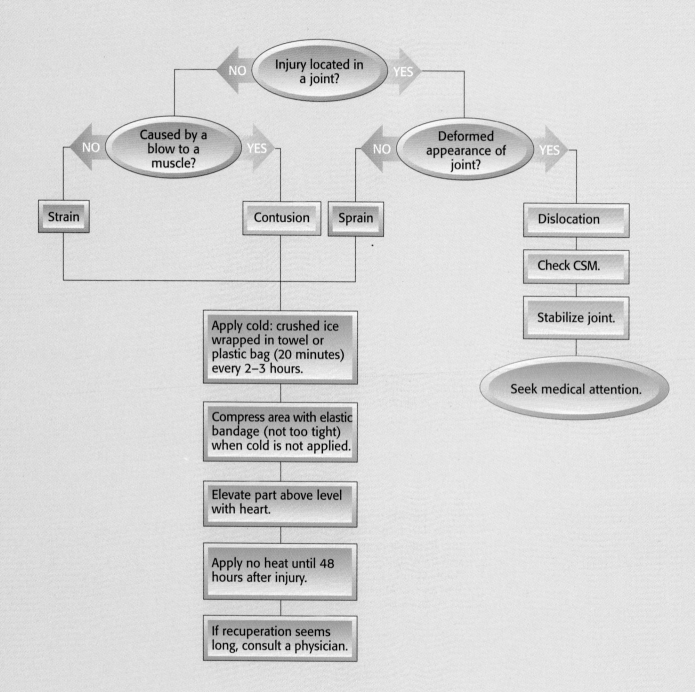

Injury located in a joint?

NO → Caused by a blow to a muscle?

NO → Strain

YES → Contusion

Sprain

YES → Deformed appearance of joint?

NO

YES → Dislocation

Apply cold: crushed ice wrapped in towel or plastic bag (20 minutes) every 2–3 hours.

Compress area with elastic bandage (not too tight) when cold is not applied.

Elevate part above level with heart.

Apply no heat until 48 hours after injury.

If recuperation seems long, consult a physician.

Check CSM.

Stabilize joint.

Seek medical attention.

- cavity, indentation, or bump that can be felt or seen
- severe weakness and loss of function of the injured part
- stiffness and pain when the victim moves the muscle

What to Do

Use the RICE procedures.

Contusions

A muscle contusion results from a blow to the muscle. Contusions are also known as bruises.

What to Look For

Any of the following signs and symptoms may occur in a muscle contusion:

- swelling
- pain and tenderness
- black-and-blue mark appearing hours later

What to Do

Use the RICE procedures.

Cramps

A cramp occurs when a muscle goes into an uncontrolled spasm and contraction, resulting in severe pain and restriction or loss of movement.

What to Do

There are many treatments for cramps. Try one or more of the following:

1. Have the victim gently stretch the affected muscle. Because a muscle cramp is an uncontrolled muscle contraction or spasm, a gradual lengthening of the muscle may help lengthen the muscle fibers and relieve the cramp.
2. Relax the muscle by applying pressure to it.
3. Apply ice to the cramped muscle to make it relax. The exception might be in a cold environment.
4. Pinch the upper lip hard (an acupressure technique) to reduce calf-muscle cramping.
5. Drink lightly salted cool water (dissolve ¼ teaspoon salt in a quart of water) or a commercial sports drink.

 CAUTION: DO NOT

- give salt tablets to a person with muscle cramps. They can cause stomach irritation, nausea, and vomiting.
- massage or rub the affected muscle. That only causes more pain and does not relieve the cramping.

RICE Procedure for Bone, Joint, and Muscle Injuries

RICE is the acronym for the first aid procedures—rest, ice, compression, elevation—for bone, joint, and muscle injuries. What is done in the first 48–72 hours following such an injury can do a lot to relieve, even prevent, aches and pains. **Treat all extremity bone, joint, and muscle injuries with the RICE procedure. In addition to RICE, fractures and dislocations should be splinted to stabilize the injured area. (See Chapter 12 for splinting techniques.)**

R = Rest

Injuries heal faster if rested. Rest means the victim stays off the injured part. Using any part of the body increases the blood circulation to that area, which can cause more swelling to an injured part. For the lower extremities, crutches may be considered.

I = Ice

An ice pack should be applied to the injured area for 20 to 30 minutes every 2 or 3 hours during the first 24 to 48 hours. Skin being treated with cold passes through four stages: cold, burning, aching, and numbness. When the skin becomes numb, usually in 20 to 30 minutes, remove the ice pack. After removing the ice pack, compress the injured part with an elastic bandage and keep it elevated (the "C" and "E" of RICE).

Cold constricts the blood vessels to and in the injured area, which helps reduce the swelling and inflammation and at the same time dulls the pain and relieves muscle spasms. Cold should be applied as soon as possible after the injury—healing time often is directly related to the amount of swelling that occurs. Heat has the opposite effect when applied to fresh injuries: it increases circulation to the area and greatly increases both the swelling and the pain.

Use either of the following methods to apply cold to an injury:

- Put crushed ice (or cubes) into a double plastic bag, hot water bottle, or wet towel. Apply one layer of a wet cloth over the injury, place the ice pack on the cloth, and then use an elastic bandage to hold the ice pack in place. Ice bags can conform to the body's contours.

- Use a chemical "snap pack," a sealed pouch that contains two chemical envelopes. Squeezing the pack mixes the chemicals, producing a chemical reaction that has a cooling effect. Although they do not cool as well as other methods, snap packs are convenient to use when ice is not readily available. They lose their cooling power quickly, however, and can be used only once. Also, they may be impractical because of their expense and the danger of breakage.

 CAUTION: DO NOT

- apply an ice pack for more than 20 to 30 minutes at a time. Frostbite or nerve damage can result.

- apply an ice pack on the back outside part of the knee. Nerve damage can occur.

- place an ice pack directly on the skin. Protect the skin with a wet cloth, which conducts cold better (a dry cloth insulates the injury from the cold).

- apply cold if the victim has a history of circulatory disease, Raynaud's syndrome (spasms in the arteries of the extremities that reduce circulation), or abnormal sensitivity to cold, or if the injured part has been frostbitten previously.

- stop using an ice pack too soon. A common mistake is too early use of heat, which will result in swelling and pain. Use an ice pack 3 to 4 times a day for the first 24 hours, preferably up to 48 hours, before applying any heat. For severe injuries, 72 hours is recommended.

C = Compression

Compression of the injured area may squeeze some fluid and debris out of the injury site. Compression limits the ability of the skin and of other tissues to expand. To try to limit internal bleeding, apply an elastic bandage to the injured area, especially the foot, ankle, knee, thigh, hand, or elbow. Fill the hollow areas with padding (e.g., sock, washcloth) before applying the elastic bandage.

Elastic bandages come in various sizes, for different body areas:

- 2-inch width, used for the wrist and hand
- 3-inch width, used for the ankle, elbow, and arm
- 4-inch width, used for the knee and leg

Start the elastic bandage several inches below the injury and wrap in an upward, overlapping (about one-half the bandage's width) spiral, starting with even and somewhat tight pressure, then gradually wrapping more loosely above the injury.

Applying compression may be the most important step in preventing swelling. The victim should wear the elastic bandage continuously for 18 to 24 hours (except when cold is applied). At night, have the victim loosen but not remove the elastic bandage.

For an ankle injury, place a horseshoe-shaped pad around the ankle knob and under the elastic bandage. The pad will permit compression of the soft tissues rather than just the bones. Wrap the bandage tightest nearest the toes and loosest above the ankle. It should be tight enough to decrease swelling but not tight enough to inhibit blood flow.

For a contusion or a strain, place a pad between the injury and the elastic bandage.

 CAUTION: DO NOT

- apply an elastic bandage too tightly. If applied too tightly, elastic bandages will restrict circulation. Stretch a new elastic bandage to about one-third its maximum length for adequate compression. Leave fingers and toes exposed so possible color change can be easily observed. Compare the toes or fingers of the injured extremity with the uninjured one. Pale skin, pain, numbness, and tingling are signs of a too tight elastic bandage. If any of these symptoms appears, immediately remove the elastic bandage. Leave the elastic bandage off until all the symptoms disappear, then rewrap the area, but less tightly. Always wrap from below the injury and move toward the heart.

1.

R = Rest
Stop using the injured part. Continued use could cause further injury, delay healing, increase pain, and stimulate bleeding. Get the victim into a comfortable position, either sitting or lying down. This slows blood flow to the injured area.

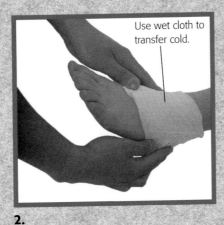

2.

Use wet cloth to transfer cold.

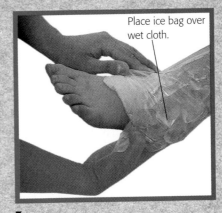

3.

Place ice bag over wet cloth.

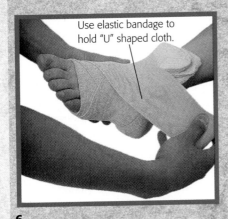

4.

Use elastic bandage to hold ice pack.

1. R = Rest
2. I ⎫
3. I ⎬ Ice
4. I ⎭
5. C ⎫
6. C ⎬ Compression
7. C ⎭
8. E = Elevation

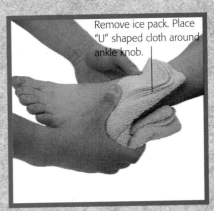

5.

Remove ice pack. Place "U" shaped cloth around ankle knob.

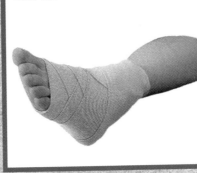

6.

Use elastic bandage to hold "U" shaped cloth.

7.

Cover heel and close to the toes.

8.

E = Elevation
Elevating the injured part is another way to decrease swelling and pain. While icing or compressing, elevate the part in whatever way is most convenient. The aim of this step is to get the injured part higher than the heart, if possible.

ANKLE INJURIES

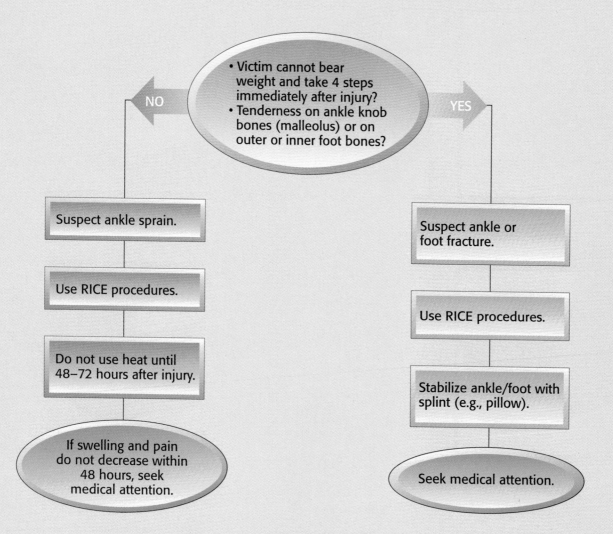

- Victim cannot bear weight and take 4 steps immediately after injury?
- Tenderness on ankle knob bones (malleolus) or on outer or inner foot bones?

NO

YES

NO branch:

Suspect ankle sprain.

Use RICE procedures.

Do not use heat until 48–72 hours after injury.

If swelling and pain do not decrease within 48 hours, seek medical attention.

YES branch:

Suspect ankle or foot fracture.

Use RICE procedures.

Stabilize ankle/foot with splint (e.g., pillow).

Seek medical attention.

E = Elevation

Gravity has an important effect on swelling. The force of gravity pulls blood and other tissue to the lower parts of the body. Once fluids get to your hands or feet, they have nowhere else to go. Thus, those parts of the body tend to swell the most. Elevating the injured area, in combination with ice and compression, limits circulation to that area, which in turn helps limit internal bleeding and minimize swelling.

It is simple to prop up an injured leg or arm to limit bleeding. Whenever possible, elevate the injured part above the level of the heart for the first 24 hours after an injury. Do not elevate an extremity if a fracture is suspected until it has been stabilized with a splint. Even then, some fractures should not be elevated.

Along with RICE, fractures and dislocations should be splinted. Chapter 12 describes splinting techniques for various parts of the body.

Blood under a Nail

When a fingernail has been crushed, blood collects under the nail. This condition usually is very painful because of the pressure of the blood pressing against the nail.

What to Do

1. Immerse the finger in ice water or apply an ice pack with the hand elevated.
2. Relieve the pressure under the injured nail by one of the following methods:
   - Using a rotary action, drill through the nail with the sharp point of a knife. This method may be painful.

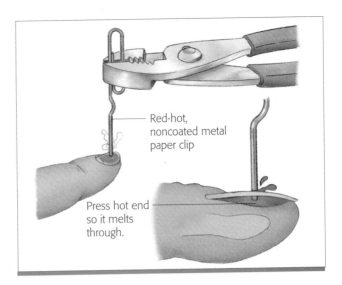

Red-hot, noncoated metal paper clip

Press hot end so it melts through.

Making a hole in a fingernail

   - Straighten the end of a metal (noncoated) paper clip or use the eye end of a sewing needle. Hold the paper clip or needle with pliers and use a match or cigarette lighter to heat it until the metal is red hot. Press the glowing end of the paper clip or needle against the nail so it melts through. Little pressure is needed. The nail has no nerves, so it is painless.

3. Apply a dressing to absorb the draining blood and to protect the injured nail.

Ring Strangulation

Sometimes a finger is so swollen that a ring cannot be removed. Ring strangulation can be a serious problem if it cuts off circulation long enough. Gangrene may result within four or five hours. Try one or more of the following methods to remove a ring:

- Lubricate the finger with grease, oil, butter, petroleum jelly, or some other slippery substance, then try to remove the ring.
- Immerse the finger in cold water or apply an ice pack for several minutes to reduce the swelling.
- Massage the finger from the tip to the hand to move the swelling; lubricate the finger again and try removing the ring.
- Smoothly wind thread around the finger, starting about an inch from the ring edge and going toward the ring, with each course touching the next. Wind smoothly and tightly right up to the

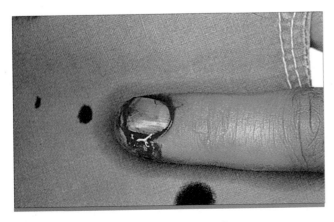

Relieve pain by releasing blood under a nail.

edge of the ring. This action will push the swelling toward the hand. Slip the end of the thread under the ring with a matchstick or toothpick, then slowly unwind the thread on the hand side of the ring. You should be able to gently twist the ring over the thread and off the finger.

- Lubricate the finger well, then pass a rubber band under the ring. Hold both ends of the rubber band and, while maintaining tension on the rubber band toward the end of the finger, pull the rubber band around and around the finger.

- Cut the narrowest part of the ring with a ring saw, jeweler's saw, ring cutter, or fine hacksaw blade. Be sure to protect the exposed portions of the finger.

- Inflate an ordinary balloon (preferably a slender, tube-shaped one) about three-fourths full. Tie the end. Insert the victim's swollen finger into the end of the balloon until the balloon evenly surrounds the entire finger. In about 15 minutes, the air pressure in the balloon should return the finger to its normal size, and the ring can be removed.

- Liberally spray window or glass cleaner onto the finger, then try to slide the ring off.

LEARNING ACTIVITIES 11

Fractures

Directions: Circle Yes if you agree with the statement, and circle No if you disagree.

Yes   No   1. For a suspected arm or leg fracture, check blood flow and nerves.

Yes   No   2. Apply cold on a suspected fracture.

Yes   No   3. A splint can help stabilize (keep in place) a fracture.

Scenario: While changing a lightbulb in a high ceiling lighting fixture, an electrician falls off a 10-foot ladder. The victim complains about a pain in his left leg. You check the left leg and find some deformity, tenderness, and swelling. What should you do?

_____

_____

_____

Dislocations and Sprains

Yes   No   1. The letters RICE represent the treatment for sprains and dislocations.

Yes   No   2. When using ice, place it directly on the skin.

Yes   No   3. Applying heat too soon to the injury is a common mistake.

Yes   No   4. An elastic bandage, if used correctly, can help control swelling in a joint.

Scenario: Your husband comes home limping and in pain. He says he twisted his ankle at work. One of his co-workers told him that it was best to "walk it out." What should you do?

_____

_____

_____

Muscle Injuries

Yes   No   1. Give salt tablets to a person suffering muscle cramps.

Yes   No   2. Apply heat initially to a muscle injury.

Yes   No   3. An elastic bandage, if used correctly, can help limit swelling.

Scenario: During a company softball game, a batter loses her grip while swinging at a pitch. The bat flies through the air and hits a nearby player hard on the thigh. While the skin is not broken, there is tenderness and some swelling. What should you do?

_____

_____

_____

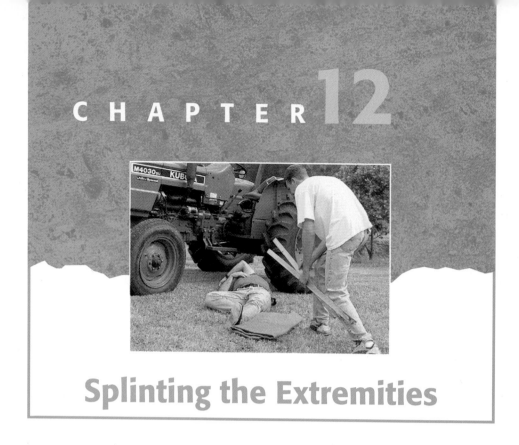

CHAPTER 12

Splinting the Extremities

Most extremity fractures are minor. The extremity is straight and medical help is nearby, so the injury can be stabilized by splinting the extremity in the position in which it was found. To *stabilize* means to use any method to hold a body part still and prevent movement. All fractures should be stabilized before a victim is moved. The reasons for splinting to stabilize an injured area are to:

- reduce pain
- prevent damage to muscle, nerves, and blood vessels
- prevent a closed fracture from becoming an open fracture
- reduce bleeding and swelling

Types of Splints

A splint is any device used to stabilize a fracture or a dislocation. Such a device can be improvised (e.g., a folded newspaper), or it can be one of several commercially available splints (e.g., SAM Splint™, air splint). Lack of a commercial splint should never prevent you from properly stabilizing an injured extremity. Many situations require ingenuity in improvisation for a first aider to render adequate care.

A rigid splint is an inflexible device attached to an extremity to maintain stability. It may be a padded board, a piece of heavy cardboard, or a SAM Splint™ molded to fit the extremity. Whatever its construction, a rigid splint must be long enough to be secured well above and below the fracture site. A soft splint, such as an air splint, is useful mainly for stabilizing fractures of the lower leg or the forearm.

A self, or anatomic, splint is almost always available. A self splint is one in which the injured body part is tied to an uninjured part (e.g., injured finger to adjacent finger, legs together, injured arm to chest).

Splinting Guidelines

All fractures and dislocations should be stabilized before the victim is moved. When in doubt, apply a splint.

CAUTION: DO NOT

- straighten dislocations or fractures of the spine, elbow, wrist, hip, or knee because of the proximity of major nerves and arteries. Instead, if the CSM (circulation-sensation-movement) is all right, splint joint injuries in the position found.

What to Do

1. Cover all open wounds, if any, with a dry, sterile dressing before applying a splint.

2. Check CSM in the extremity. If pulses are absent, try to straighten the fracture or dislocation to restore blood flow.

3. Determine what to splint by using the "rule of thirds." Imagine each long bone as being divided into thirds. If the injury is located in the upper or lower third of a bone, assume that the nearest joint is injured. Therefore, the splint should extend to stabilize the bones above and below the unstable joint; for example, for a fracture of the upper third of the tibia (shinbone), the splint must extend to include the upper leg, as well as the lower leg, because the knee is unstable.

    For a fracture of the middle third of a bone stabilize the joints above and below the fracture (e.g., wrist and elbow for fractured radius or ulna; shoulder and elbow for fractured humerus; knee and ankle for fractured tibia or fibula). An upper extremity fracture, in addition to being splinted, should be placed in an arm sling and a swathe (binder).

4. If two first aiders are present, one should support the injury site and minimize movement of the extremity until splinting is completed.

5. When possible, place splint materials on both sides of the injured part, especially when two bones are involved (e.g., radius/ulna or tibia/fibula). This "sandwich splint" prevents rotation of the injured extremity and keeps the two bones from touching. With rigid splints, use extra padding in natural body hollows and around any deformities.

6. Apply splints firmly but not so tight that blood flow into an extremity is affected. Check CSM before and periodically after the splint is applied. If the pulse disappears, loosen the splint enough so you can feel the pulse. Leave the fingers or toes exposed so CSM can be checked easily.

7. Use RICE on the injured part. When practicable, elevation of the injured extremity after stabilization promotes drainage from the limb by gravity and reduces swelling. *Do not, however, apply ice packs if a pulse is absent.*

Most fractures do not require rapid transportation. An exception is an arm or a leg without a pulse, which means insufficient blood flow to that extremity. In that case, *immediate* medical attention is necessary.

Arm Sling: Shoulder and Clavicle Injuries

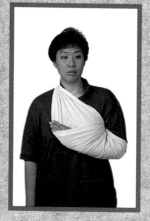
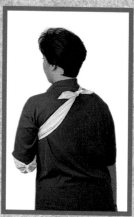

Upper Arm (Humerus)

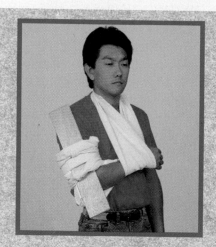

Arm Sling and Swathe for Upper Extremity Injuries

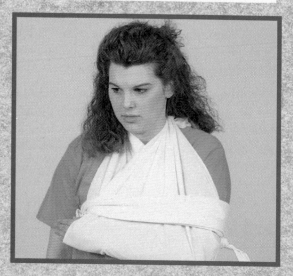

Forearm (Radius/Ulna)

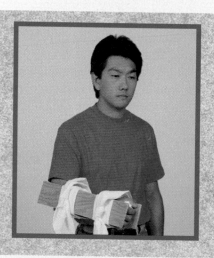

Fingers and Hand (Position of Function)

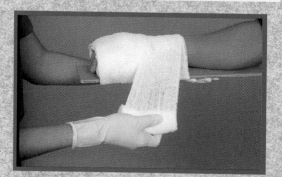

Elbow in Bent Position

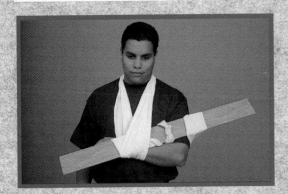

Knee in Bent Position

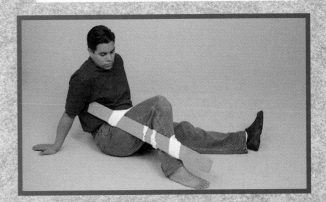

Elbow in Straight Position

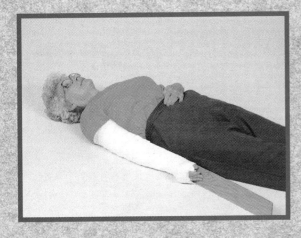

Knee in Straight Position

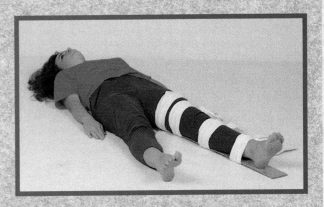

Lower Leg (Tibia/Fibula)

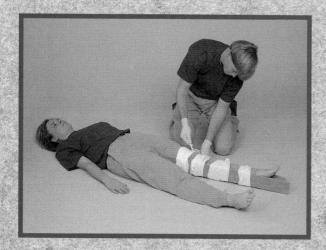

Thigh (Femur)

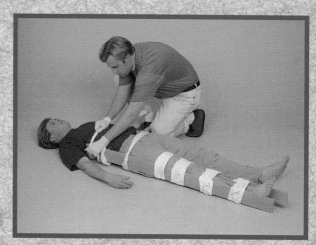

Ankle/Foot

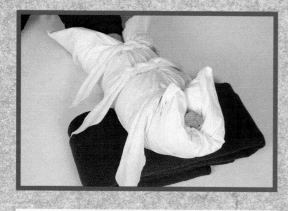

Self-Splint: Leg

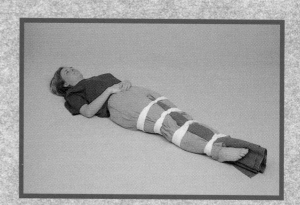

Self-Splint: Fingers/Toes

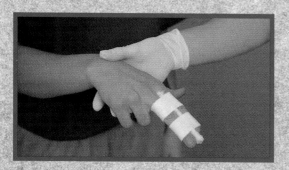

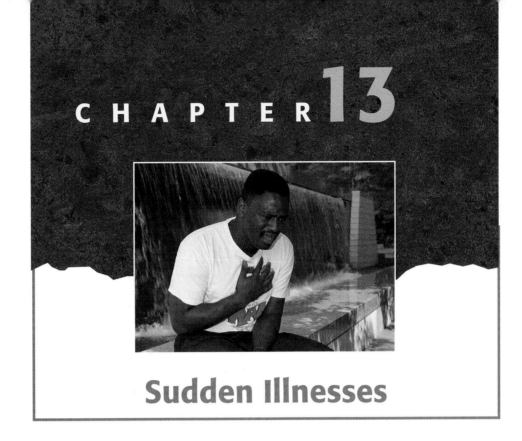

CHAPTER 13

Sudden Illnesses

Heart Attack

A heart attack occurs when the blood supply to part of the heart muscle is severely reduced or stopped. That happens when one of the coronary arteries (the arteries that supply blood to the heart muscle) is blocked by an obstruction or a spasm.

What to Look For

Heart attacks are difficult to determine. Because medical care at the onset of a heart attack is vital to survival and the quality of recovery, if you suspect a heart attack for any reason, seek medical attention *at once*.

The American Heart Association lists the following as possible signs and symptoms of a heart attack:

- uncomfortable pressure, fullness, squeezing, or pain in the center of the chest that lasts more than a few minutes or that goes away and comes back
- pain spreading to the shoulders, neck, or arms
- chest discomfort with lightheadedness, fainting, sweating, nausea, or shortness of breath

Not all these warning signs occur in every heart attack. It is difficult to determine if someone is having a heart attack. Many victims will deny that they might be experiencing something as serious as a heart attack. Don't take "no" for an answer. Delay can seriously increase the risk of major damage. Insist on taking prompt action.

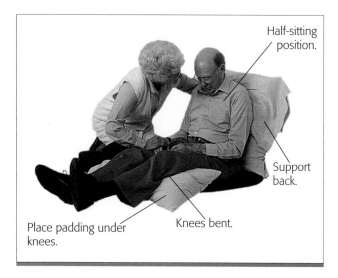

Half-sitting position.

Support back.

Knees bent.

Place padding under knees.

Help the victim into a relaxed position to ease strain on heart.

What to Do

1. Call the EMS or get to the nearest hospital emergency department that offers 24-hour emergency cardiac care.

2. Monitor the ABCs. Give CPR if necessary.

3. Help the victim to the least painful position, usually sitting with legs up and bent at the knees. Loosen clothing around the neck and midriff. Be calm and reassuring.

4. Determine if the victim is known to have coronary heart disease and is using nitroglycerin. Nitroglycerin tablets or spray under the tongue or nitroglycerin ointment on the skin may relieve chest pain. Nitroglycerin dilates the coronary arteries, which increases blood flow to the heart muscle, and lowers blood pressure and dilates the veins, which decreases the work of the heart and the heart muscle's need for oxygen.

   Caution: Because nitroglycerin lowers blood pressure, the victim should be sitting or lying down. Nitroglycerin normally may be repeated for a total of three doses in 10 minutes if the first dose does not relieve the pain. Keep in mind, though, that the victim may have already taken some nitroglycerin. Also, nitroglycerin is prescribed in different strengths—three tablets of one strength may be a mild dose, while three tablets of another strength may be a very high dose.

5. If the victim is unresponsive, check the ABCs and start CPR if needed.

Angina

Chest pain called angina pectoris can result from coronary heart disease just as a heart attack does. Angina happens when the heart muscle does not get as much blood as it needs (which means a lack of oxygen).

Angina is brought on by physical exertion, exposure to cold, emotional stress, or the ingestion of food. It seldom lasts longer than 10 minutes and almost always is relieved by nitroglycerin. (In contrast, chest pain from a heart attack is as likely to happen at rest as during activity; the pain lasts longer than 10 minutes and is not relieved by nitroglycerin.)

Stroke (Brain Attack)

A stroke, or cerebrovascular accident (CVA), occurs when blood vessels that deliver oxygen-rich blood to the brain rupture or become plugged, so part of the brain does not get the blood flow it needs. Deprived of oxygen, nerve cells in the affected area of the brain cannot function and die within minutes. Because dead brain cells are not replaced, the devastating effects of strokes often are permanent.

Transient ischemic attacks (TIAs) are closely associated with CVAs. Because TIAs have many of the same signs and symptoms, they often are confused with strokes. The main difference between a TIA and a stroke is that the symptoms of TIA are transient, lasting from several minutes (75 percent last less than five minutes) to several hours, with a return to normal neurologic function. TIAs are "mini-strokes." A TIA should be considered a serious warning sign of a potential stroke—about one-third of all TIA cases will suffer a CVA two to five years after their first TIA. Any signs and symptoms of a TIA should be reported to a physician.

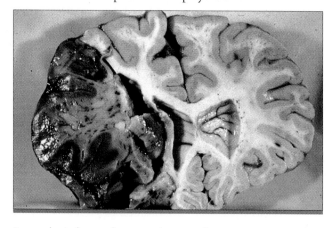

Severe brain hemorrhage causing a stroke

What to Look For

- weakness, numbness, or paralysis of the face, an arm, or a leg on one side of the body
- blurred or decreased vision, especially in one eye
- problems speaking or understanding
- dizziness or loss of balance
- sudden, severe, and unexplained headache
- deviation of the eyes from PEARL (**P**upils **E**qual **A**nd **R**eactive to **L**ight), which may mean the brain is being affected by lack of oxygen

What to Do

First aid for a stroke victim is limited to supportive care:

1. If the victim is unresponsive, check the ABCs.
2. Call the EMS.
3. Lay the victim down with the head and shoulders slightly elevated, to reduce blood pressure on the brain. Place a victim who is unresponsive but breathing in the recovery position, which is on the left side with the chin extended (to keep the airway open and to permit secretions and vomit to drain from the mouth).

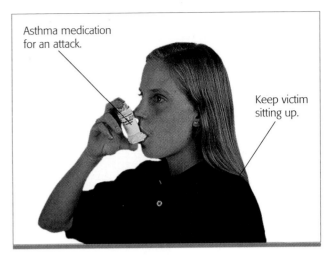

Asthma medication for an attack.

Keep victim sitting up.

Keep an asthma victim comfortable.

2. Keep the victim in a comfortable upright position that makes it easier to breathe.
3. Ask the victim about any asthma medication he or she may be using. Most asthma sufferers will have some form of asthma medication, usually administered through doctor-prescribed, hand-held inhalers.
4. If the victim does not respond well to his or her inhaled medication or is having an extreme asthma attack (known as status asthmaticus), seek medical attention immediately.

 CAUTION: DO NOT

- **give a stroke victim anything to drink or eat. The throat may be paralyzed, which restricts swallowing.**

 CAUTION: DO NOT

- **wait too long to get medical help for the victim of a severe asthma attack.**

Asthma
What to Look For

- coughing
- cyanosis (bluish skin color)
- inability to speak in complete sentences without pausing for breath
- nostrils flaring with each breath
- wheezing (high-pitched whistling sound during breathing)

What to Do

1. Check the ABCs (airway open, breathing, and pulse).

Hyperventilation

Fast, deep breathing is common during psychological stress.

What to Look For

- dizziness or lightheadedness
- numbness
- tingling of the hands and feet
- shortness of breath
- breathing rates faster than 40 per minute

What to Do

1. Calm and reassure the victim.

2. Encourage the victim to breathe slowly, using the abdominal muscles: inhale through the nose, hold the full inhalation for several seconds, then exhale slowly through pursed lips.
3. Do not have the victim breathe into a paper bag.

Fainting

Most fainting is associated with decreased blood flow to the brain. The decreased blood flow may be caused by low blood sugar (hypoglycemia), slow heart rate (vagal reaction, in which the vagus nerve, which slows the heart rate, is overstimulated by fright, anxiety, drugs, fatigue), heart-rhythm disturbances, dehydration, heat exhaustion, anemia, or bleeding.

Sitting or standing for a long time without moving, especially in a hot environment, can cause blood to pool in dilated vessels. That results in a loss of effective circulating blood volume, which causes the blood pressure to drop. As the brain's blood flow decreases, the person loses consciousness and collapses.

What to Look For

A person who is about to faint usually will have one or more of the following signs and symptoms:

- dizziness
- weakness
- seeing spots
- visual blurring
- nausea
- pale skin
- sweating

What to Do

If a person appears about to faint,

1. Prevent the person from falling.
2. Help the person lie down and raise the legs 8–12 inches. This position increases venous blood flow back to the heart, which in turn pumps more blood to the brain.

If fainting has happened or is anticipated,

1. Lay the victim down and raise the legs 8–12 inches.
2. Loosen tight clothing and belts.

3. If the victim has fallen, check for any sign of injury. If nothing is suspected, have the victim sit for a while and, when able to swallow, drink cool, sweetened liquids, and slowly regain an upright posture.
4. Fresh air and a cold, wet cloth for the face usually aid recovery.

CAUTION: DO NOT

- splash or pour water on the victim's face.
- use smelling salts or ammonia inhalants.
- slap the victim's face in an attempt to revive him or her.
- give the victim anything to drink until he or she has fully recovered and can swallow.

Most fainting episodes are not serious, and the victim regains consciousness quickly. Seek medical attention, however, if the victim

- is over 40 years old
- has had repeated attacks of unconsciousness
- does not waken in four or five minutes
- loses consciousness while sitting or lying down
- faints for no apparent reason

Seizures

A seizure is the result of an abnormal stimulation of the brain's cells. A variety of medical conditions increase the instability or irritability of the brain and can lead to seizures, including the following:

- epilepsy
- heatstroke
- poisoning
- electric shock
- hypoglycemia
- high fever in children
- brain injury, tumor, or stroke
- alcohol withdrawal, drug abuse/overdose

Epilepsy is not a mental illness, and it is not a sign of low intelligence. It also is not contagious. Between seizures, a person with epilepsy can function as normally as a nonepileptic.

What to Do

The Epilepsy Foundation of America lists the following first aid procedures for seizures:

1. Cushion the victim's head; take away items that could cause injury if the person bumped into them.
2. Loosen any tight neckwear.
3. Turn the victim onto his or her left side.
4. Look for a medical-alert tag (bracelet or necklace).
5. As the seizure ends, offer your help. Most seizures in people with epilepsy are not medical emergencies. They end after a minute or two without harm and usually do not require medical attention.
6. Call EMS if any of the following exists:
   - A seizure happens to someone who is not known to have epilepsy (e.g., there is no "epilepsy" or "seizure disorder" identification). It could be a sign of serious illness.
   - A seizure lasts more than five minutes.
   - The victim is slow to recover, has a second seizure, or has difficulty breathing afterward.
   - The victim is pregnant or has another medical condition.
   - There are any signs of injury or illnesses.

CAUTION: DO NOT

- give the victim anything to eat or drink.
- hold the victim down.
- put anything between the victim's teeth during the seizure.
- throw any liquid on the victim's face or into the mouth.
- move the victim to another place.

Diabetic Emergencies

Diabetes is a condition in which insulin, a hormone produced by the pancreas that helps the body use the energy in food, is either lacking or ineffective. The function of insulin is to take sugar from the blood and carry it into the cells to be used. When excess sugar remains in the blood, the body cells must rely on fat as fuel. Blood sugar is a major body fuel, and when it cannot be used, it builds up in the blood and overflows into the urine and passes out of the body unused—the body loses an important source of fuel. Diabetes develops. Diabetes is not contagious.

There are two types of diabetes:

- *Type I: juvenile-onset or insulin-dependent* diabetes. Type I diabetics require external (not made by the body) insulin to allow sugar to pass from the blood into cells. When deprived of external insulin, the diabetic becomes quite ill.
- *Type II: adult-onset or non–insulin-dependent* diabetes. Type II diabetics tend to be overweight. They are not dependent on external insulin to allow sugar into cells. However, if their insulin level is low, the lack of sugar in the cells increases sugar production and sugar in the blood to very high levels. That causes glucose to spill into the urine, which draws fluid with it, resulting in dehydration.

The body is continuously balancing sugar and insulin. Too much insulin and not enough sugar leads to low blood sugar, possibly insulin shock. Too much sugar and not enough insulin leads to high blood sugar, possibly diabetic coma.

Low Blood Sugar

Very low blood sugar, called hypoglycemia, is sometimes referred to as an "insulin reaction." This condition can be caused by too much insulin, too little or delayed food, exercise, alcohol, or any combination of these factors.

The American Diabetes Association lists the following signs and symptoms of insulin reaction and hypoglycemia as diabetic emergencies requiring first aid:

- sudden onset
- staggering, poor coordination
- anger, bad temper
- pale color
- confusion, disorientation
- sudden hunger
- excessive sweating
- trembling
- eventual unconsciousness

What to Do

Give sugar if all are present:

- The victim is a known diabetic, and

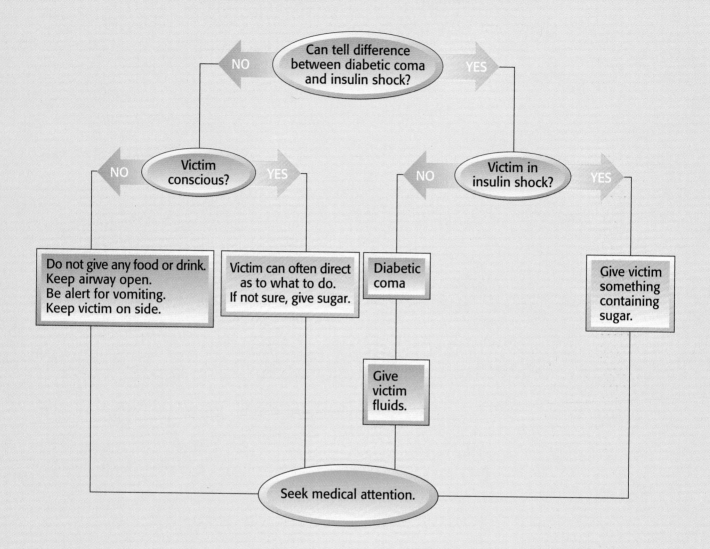

Can tell difference between diabetic coma and insulin shock?

NO → **Victim conscious?**

NO → Do not give any food or drink. Keep airway open. Be alert for vomiting. Keep victim on side.

YES → Victim can often direct as to what to do. If not sure, give sugar.

YES → **Victim in insulin shock?**

NO → Diabetic coma → Give victim fluids.

YES → Give victim something containing sugar.

Seek medical attention.

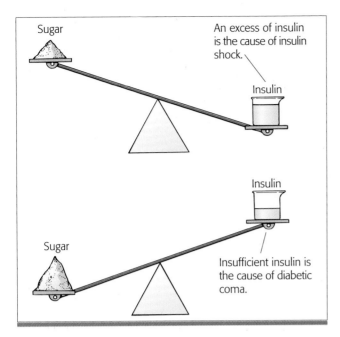

Sugar

An excess of insulin is the cause of insulin shock.

Insulin

Insulin

Sugar

Insufficient insulin is the cause of diabetic coma.

Diabetic emergencies

High Blood Sugar

Hyperglycemia is the opposite of hypoglycemia. Hyperglycemia occurs when the body has too much sugar in the blood. This condition may be caused by insufficient insulin, overeating, inactivity, illness, stress, or a combination of these factors.

The American Diabetes Association lists the following signs and symptoms of diabetic coma and hyperglycemia as diabetic emergencies requiring first aid:

- gradual onset
- drowsiness
- extreme thirst
- very frequent urination
- flushed skin
- vomiting
- fruity breath odor
- heavy breathing
- eventual unconsciousness

What to Do

1. If you are uncertain whether victim has high or low blood-sugar level, give the person sugar-containing food or drink.
2. If improvement is not seen in 15 minutes, take the victim to the hospital.

- The victim's mental status is altered, and
- The victim is awake enough to swallow.

1. Give victim sugar-containing food, such as soda, candy, milk, or fruit juice. Do not use diet drinks—they do not contain sugar.
2. If improvement is not seen in 15 minutes, take the person to a hospital.

Sudden Illness

Directions: Circle Yes if you agree with the statement, and circle No if you disagree.

Yes No 1. Heart attack victims experience the least amount of chest pain when lying down.

Yes No 2. When taking doctor-prescribed nitroglycerine for chest pain, the person should be sitting or lying down.

Yes No 3. A stroke victim should have his or her head slightly raised.

Yes No 4. Most asthma victims will usually have a doctor-prescribed inhaler.

Yes No 5. A victim who is breathing fast (hyperventilation) should be encouraged to breathe slowly by holding inhaled air for several seconds, then exhaling slowly.

Yes No 6. Splash or sprinkle water on a person who has fainted.

Yes No 7. Have a fainted victim inhale smelling salts or ammonia inhalants.

Yes No 8. Place a strong stick or similar object between a seizure victim's teeth.

Yes No 9. A person having seizures always requires medical attention.

Yes No 10. If in doubt about whether a victim has an insulin reaction or is in a diabetic coma, give sugar to a responsive victim who can swallow.

Yes No 11. During a diabetic emergency and if improvement is not seen in 15 minutes, seek medical attention for the victim.

Scenario #1: A 50-year-old co-worker complains about chest pain. He says that it started about an hour ago and has not let up since. He is sure that it is just a little indigestion and feels silly about talking about it. He says the pain feels like "something pressing on my chest," and he feels nauseous. What should you do?

_____

_____

Scenario #2: You are working in an office cubicle next to a co-worker who suddenly collapses. You rush to help and find him confused, with numbness and paralysis on one side. Another co-worker said that he had complained of a severe headache earlier. What should you do?

_____

_____

Scenario #3: During a first aid training video showing a bloodied victim, a young man suddenly falls from his chair to the floor. He is breathing and has a pulse, but is unresponsive. No other injuries from the fall are detected. What should you do?

_____

_____

Scenario #4: You see some of your co-workers holding down another employee on the floor. They are trying to force a couple of pencils between her teeth. The person is unresponsive and is having severe muscle jerks. What should you do?

_____

_____

Scenario #5: After work, the car-pool driver is driving fast and erratically. When she stops to let her first rider out, she just sits in the car staring ahead. She then slumps over onto the steering wheel. Her skin is cold and sweaty. You are aware the driver is diabetic. What should you do?

_____

_____

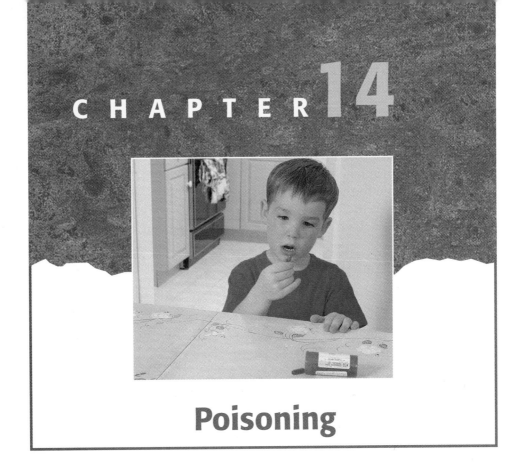

CHAPTER 14

Poisoning

Ingested (Swallowed) Poison

Fortunately, most poison ingestions happen with products of low toxicity or with amounts so small that severe poisoning rarely occurs. However, the potential for severe or fatal poisoning is always present.

What to Look For

- abdominal pain and cramping
- nausea or vomiting
- diarrhea
- burns, odor, stains around and in mouth
- drowsiness or unconsciousness
- poison containers nearby

What to Do

1. Determine critical information:
    - Age and size of the victim?
    - What was swallowed?
    - How much was swallowed (e.g., a "taste," half a bottle, a dozen tablets)?
    - When was it swallowed?
2. If a corrosive or caustic (i.e., acid or alkali) substance was swallowed, immediately dilute it by having the victim drink at least 1–2 eight-ounce glasses of water or milk. (*Cold* milk or water tends to absorb heat better than room-temperature or warmer liquids.)

CAUTION: DO NOT

- give water or milk to dilute other poisons unless instructed to do so by a poison control center. Fluids may dissolve a dry poison (e.g., tablets or capsules) more rapidly and fill up the stomach, forcing stomach contents (i.e., the poison) into the small intestine, where poisons are absorbed faster.

3. For a responsive victim, call a poison control center *immediately*. Some poisons do not cause harm until hours later, while others damage immediately. More than 70 percent of poisonings can be treated through instructions taken over the telephone from a poison control center. The center also will advise you if medical attention is warranted. Poison control centers routinely follow up calls to check whether additional symptoms or unexpected effects are occurring. The inside front covers of telephone directories contain the poison control center's number.

4. For an unresponsive victim, or if the poison control center number is unknown, call 911 or the local emergency number. Monitor the ABCs often.

5. Place the victim on his or her *left* side to position the end of the stomach where it enters the small intestine (pylorus) straight up. Gravity will delay (by as much as two hours) advancement of the poison into the small intestine, where absorption into the victim's circulatory system is faster. The side position also helps prevent aspiration (inhalation) into the lungs if vomiting begins.

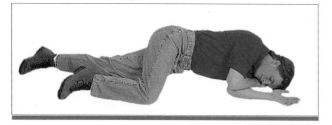

The left-side position delays the poison from advancing into the small intestine.

6. Induce vomiting *only* if a poison control center or a physician advises it. Inducing must be done within 30 minutes of swallowing.

    If you are instructed by a poison control center or a physician to induce vomiting, use syrup of ipecac. It can be purchased without a prescription and is easily given. Follow the directions carefully. Ipecac will not work unless sufficient water also is given.

7. Give activated charcoal, the single most effective agent for most swallowed poisons. Activated charcoal acts like a sponge and binds and keeps the poison in the digestive system, thus preventing absorption of the poison into the blood.

    While activated charcoal may appear similar to burnt-toast scrapings and charcoal briquettes, they *cannot* be used interchangeably.

    Not all chemicals, however, are absorbed well by activated charcoal, including acids and alkalies (e.g., bleach, ammonia), potassium, iron, alcohol, methanol, kerosene, cyanide, malathion, and ferrous sulfate.

    Major drawbacks of activated charcoal are its grittiness and its appearance. Trying to improve the taste or consistency by adding chocolate syrup, sherbet, ice cream, milk, or other flavoring agents only decreases the charcoal's binding capacity. Placing the charcoal mixture in an opaque container and having the victim sip it through a straw makes it more palatable. First aiders should give only the pre-mixed form.

    Although activated charcoal is an inexpensive, safe, and effective means for decreasing poison absorption, pharmacies do not routinely stock it.

8. Save poison containers, plants, and the victim's vomit to help medical personnel identify the poison.

Alcohol and Drug Emergencies
Alcohol Intoxication

Helping an intoxicated person is often difficult since the individual may be belligerent and combative. Also, personal hygiene is sometimes less than optimal. However, it is important that alcohol abusers be helped and not just labeled as "drunks." Their condition may be quite serious, even life threatening.

SWALLOWED POISON

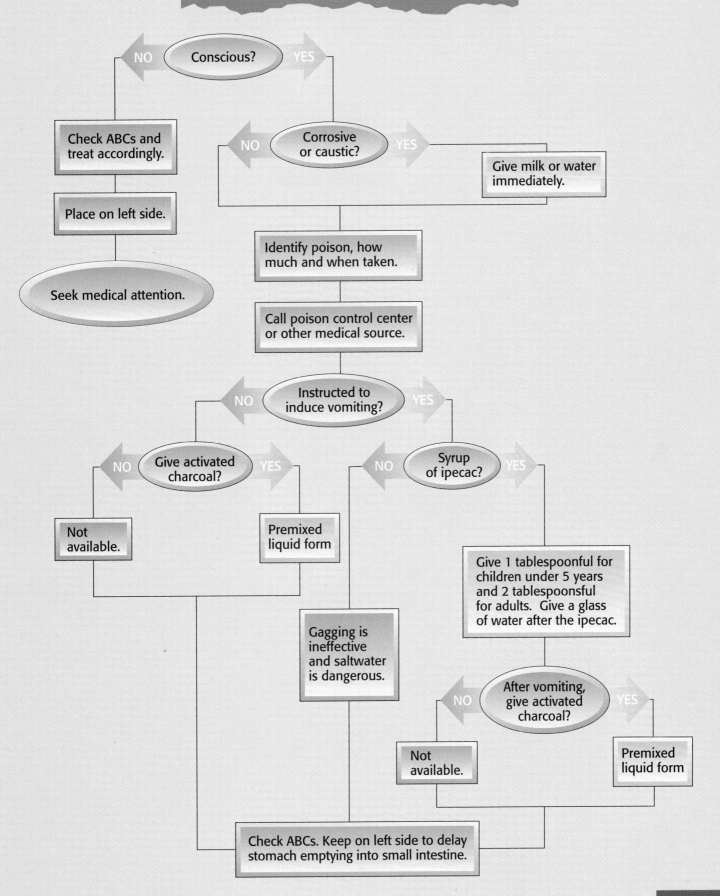

Conscious?

NO → Check ABCs and treat accordingly. → Place on left side. → Seek medical attention.

YES → **Corrosive or caustic?**

- YES → Give milk or water immediately.
- NO → Identify poison, how much and when taken. → Call poison control center or other medical source. → **Instructed to induce vomiting?**

Instructed to induce vomiting?

NO → **Give activated charcoal?**
- NO → Not available.
- YES → Premixed liquid form
- Gagging is ineffective and saltwater is dangerous.

YES → **Syrup of ipecac?**
- NO → (Gagging is ineffective and saltwater is dangerous.)
- YES → Give 1 tablespoonful for children under 5 years and 2 tablespoonsful for adults. Give a glass of water after the ipecac. → **After vomiting, give activated charcoal?**
  - NO → Not available.
  - YES → Premixed liquid form

Check ABCs. Keep on left side to delay stomach emptying into small intestine.

What to Look For

The following signs are indicators of alcohol intoxication. (Some of these symptoms can also mean illness or injury other than alcohol abuse, such as diabetes or heat injury.)

- the odor of alcohol on a person's breath or clothing
- unsteady, staggering walking
- slurred speech and the inability to carry on a conversation
- nausea and vomiting
- flushed face

What to Do

First aid for an intoxicated person includes these steps:

1. Look for any injuries. Alcohol can mask pain.
2. Check the ABCDs and treat accordingly.
3. If the intoxicated person is lying down, place him or her in the recovery (left-side) position, to reduce the likelihood of vomiting and aspiration of vomit and to delay absorption. Be sure to check that the victim is breathing and does not have a spine injury before you move him or her. The recovery position can be used for both responsive and unresponsive persons.
4. Call the poison control center for advice or the local emergency number for help. It may be best to let EMS personnel decide if the police should be alerted.
5. If the victim becomes violent, leave the scene and find a safe place until police arrive.
6. Provide emotional support.
7. Assume that an injured or unresponsive victim has a spine injury and needs to be stabilized against movement. Because of decreased pain perception, an intoxicated victim cannot be assessed reliably. If you suspect a spine injury, wait for the EMS to arrive. They have the proper equipment and training to stabilize and move a victim.
8. Since many intoxicated individuals have been exposed to the cold, suspect hypothermia and move the person to a warm environment. Remove wet clothing and cover the individual with warm blankets. Handle a hypothermic victim gently, since rough handling could induce a heart attack.

CAUTION: DO NOT

- let an intoxicated person sleep on his or her back.
- leave an intoxicated person alone.
- try to handle a hostile drunk by yourself. Find a safe place, then call the police for help.

Drugs

What to Do

1. Check the ABCDs.
2. Call the poison control center for advice or the EMS for help.
3. Check for injuries.
4. Keep the person on the *left* side to reduce the likelihood of vomiting and aspiration of vomit and to delay absorption.
5. Provide reassurance and emotional support.
6. If the person becomes violent, find a safe place until the police arrive. Let law enforcement officers handle dangerous situations.
7. Seek medical attention.

Carbon Monoxide Poisoning

Carbon monoxide (CO) victims often are unaware of its presence. The gas is invisible, tasteless, odorless, and nonirritating. It is produced by the incomplete burning of organic material such as gasoline, wood, paper, charcoal, coal, and natural gas.

What to Look For

It is difficult to tell if a person is a CO victim. Sometimes, a complaint of having the "flu" is really a symptom of CO poisoning. Although many symptoms of CO poisoning resemble those of the flu, there are differences. For example, CO poisoning does not cause low-grade fever or generalized aching or involve the lymph nodes.

The following conditions are earmarks of possible CO poisoning:

- The symptoms come and go.
- The symptoms worsen or improve in certain places or at certain times of the day.
- People around the victim have similar symptoms.
- Pets seem ill.

The signs and symptoms of CO poisoning are as follows:

- headache
- ringing in the ears (tinnitus)
- chest pain (angina)
- muscle weakness
- nausea and vomiting
- dizziness and visual changes (blurred or double vision)
- unconsciousness
- respiratory and cardiac arrest

What to Do

1. Remove the victim from the toxic environment and into fresh air *immediately*.
2. Call the EMS, which will be able to give the victim 100 percent oxygen, improving oxygenation and disassociating the linkage between the CO and the hemoglobin.

3. Monitor the ABCs.
4. Place an unresponsive victim on one side.
5. Seek medical attention. All suspected CO victims should obtain a blood test to determine the level of CO.

Poison Ivy, Poison Oak, and Poison Sumac

Most people cannot identify these irritating plants. A helpful method of identifying these plants is the "black-spot test." When the sap is exposed to the air, it turns brown in a matter of minutes and by the next day is black.

What to Do

1. For those who know they have contacted a poisonous plant, decontaminate the skin as soon as possible (within five minutes for sensitive

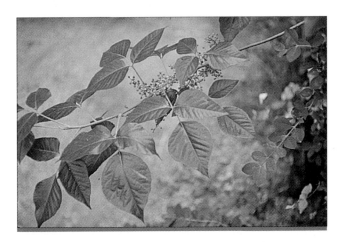

Poison ivy, found in all 48 contiguous U.S. states

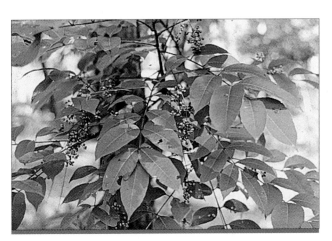

Poison sumac

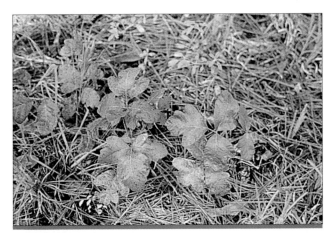

Poison oak

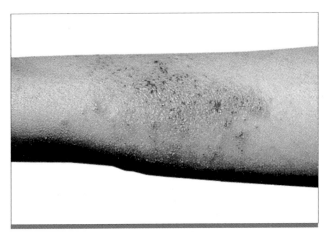

Poison ivy dermatitis

people, up to one hour for moderately sensitive individuals). (Most victims do not know about their contact until several hours or days later, when the itching and rash begin.) Use soap and cold water to clean the skin of the oily resin or apply rubbing (isopropyl) alcohol liberally (not in swab-type dabs). If too little isopropyl alcohol is used, the oil will actually be spread to another site and enlarge the injury. Other solvents (e.g., paint thinner, gasoline) can be used, but they are hard on the skin. Rinse with water to remove the solubilized material. Water removes urushiol (plant resin) from the skin, oxidizes and inactivates it, and does not penetrate the skin as do solvents.

2. For the mild stage, have the victim soak in a lukewarm bath sprinkled with one to two cups of colloidal oatmeal (e.g., Aveeno™) (colloidal oatmeal makes a tub slick, so take appropriate precautions) or apply any of the following:

- wet compresses soaked with Burow's solution (aluminum acetate) for 20–30 minutes three or four times a day
- calamine lotion (calamine ointment if the skin becomes dry and cracked) or zinc oxide
- baking soda paste, which is one teaspoon of water mixed with three teaspoons of baking soda

3. For the mild to moderate stage, care for the skin as you would for the mild stage and use a physician-prescribed corticosteroid ointment.

4. For the severe stage, care for the skin as you would for the mild and moderate stages and use a physician-prescribed oral corticosteroid (e.g., prednisone). Apply a topical corticosteroid ointment or cream, cover it with a transparent plastic wrap, and lightly bind the area with an elastic or self-adhering bandage.

LEARNING ACTIVITIES 14

Poisoning

Directions: Circle Yes if you agree with the statement, and circle No if you disagree.

Yes No 1. If a corrosive or caustic substance was swallowed, immediately dilute it by having the victim drink water or milk.

Yes No 2. For a poisoned victim, call a poison control center immediately.

Yes No 3. Induce vomiting with ipecac syrup only if advised by a poison control center or a doctor.

Yes No 4. Place a swallowed poisoned victim on his or her left side to delay having the poison go into the small intestine.

Yes No 5. Do NOT let an intoxicated person sleep on his or her back.

Yes No 6. If an intoxicated or drugged person becomes violent, leave the scene and let law enforcement officers handle the situation.

Yes No 7. Seek medical attention for all carbon monoxide victims.

Yes No 8. Calamine lotion can help relieve itching caused by poison ivy, oak, or sumac.

Yes No 9. Some cases of poison ivy, oak, or sumac require medical attention.

Scenario #1: You find your 2-year-old son, Scott, vomiting. You notice the top of a nearby medicine container is off. The label on the container indicates that the medicine is your visiting mother's. You realize that Scott must have swallowed some of the highly potent medicine. What should you do?

_____

_____

Scenario #2: While at one of your boss's parties, one of the guests becomes quite drunk. He has vomited and has become unresponsive. What should you do?

_____

_____

Scenario #3: A 25-year-old co-worker seems to be "freaking out." Another co-worker says she saw the victim take some "pills." After yelling and screaming inside the office, she finally calms down enough to tell you that she took some drugs. What should you do?

_____

_____

Scenario #4: A co-worker has been moving various items in a storage room and left a truck's motor running. All of the room's windows and doors have been closed because of the subfreezing outside temperatures. Other co-workers found him and have moved him to fresh air just as you arrive. What should you do?

_____

_____

Scenario #5: While weeding around a vacant lot, you pull up a batch of weeds with shiny leaves in clusters of three. You finish the job about an hour later. The next morning your arms are itching, and you notice a rash beginning to appear. What should you do?

_____

_____

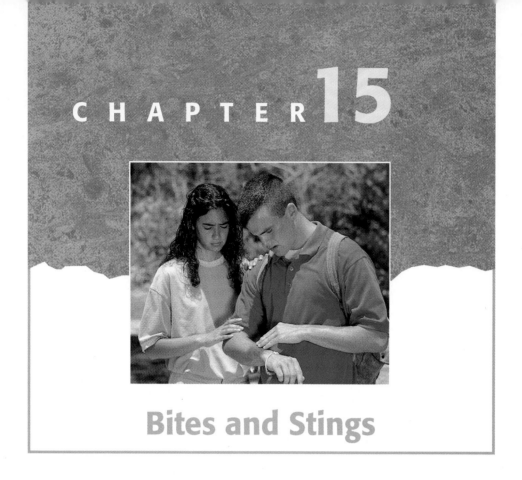

CHAPTER 15

Bites and Stings

Animal Bites

It is estimated that one of every two Americans will be bitten at some time by an animal* or by another person. Dogs are responsible for about 80 percent of all animal-bite injuries.

Rabies

A virus found in warm-blooded animals causes rabies and spreads from one animal to another in the saliva, usually through a bite or by licking.

Consider an animal as possibly rabid if any of the following applies:

- The animal attacked unprovoked.
- The animal acted strangely, that is, out of character (e.g., a usually friendly dog is aggressive, or a wild fox seems docile and "friendly").
- The animal was a high-risk species (skunk, raccoon, or bat).

What to Do

1. If the victim was bitten in the United States (except for the area along the border with Mexico) by a healthy domestic dog or cat, the animal should be confined and observed for 10 days for any illness. If the offending animal is a stray or unwanted dog or cat, it should be killed immediately and its head submitted for rabies examination. If feasible, only a veterinarian should kill an animal (domesticated or wild) and decapitate it for sending

*As it is commonly interpreted, the term *animal bite* in this section refers to a bite by a mammal, not by an insect or reptile.

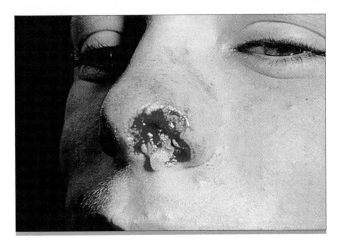

Dog bite

1. If the wound is not bleeding heavily, wash it with soap and water (under the pressure from a faucet) for 5 to 10 minutes. Avoid scrubbing, which can traumatize tissues.
2. Rinse the wound thoroughly with running water under pressure.
3. Control bleeding with direct pressure.
4. Cover the wound with a sterile dressing. Do *not* close the wound with tape or butterfly bandages. That traps bacteria in the wound, increasing the chance of infection.
5. Seek medical attention for possible further wound cleaning, a tetanus shot, and sutures applied to close the wound.

the head to a laboratory. If the animal is dead, transport the entire body; do *not* attempt decapitation (precautions must be taken to prevent exposure to potentially infected tissues and saliva).

Report animal bites to the police or animal control officers; they should be the ones to capture the animal for observation. If the dog or cat escapes and is not suspected to be rabid, consult local public health officials.

If the victim was bitten in the United States by a skunk, raccoon, bat, fox, or other mammal, it should be considered a rabies exposure and treatment started *immediately*. The only exception is when the bite occurred in a part of the continental United States known to be free of rabies. If the wild animal is captured, it should be killed and its head shipped to a qualified laboratory immediately.

2. Clean the wound with a soap solution, rinse it with water under pressure.
3. Stop the bleeding and give wound care.
4. Seek medical attention for further wound cleaning and a possible tetanus shot. The physician will determine if sutures are needed to close the wound. If needed, a vaccination against rabies will be started.

Human Bites

The human mouth contains a wide range of bacteria, so the chance of infection is greater from a human bite than from bites of other warm-blooded animals.

Snakebites

Only four snake species in the United States are venomous: rattlesnakes (which account for about 65 percent of all venomous snakebites and nearly all the snakebite deaths in the United States), copperheads, water moccasins (also known as cottonmouths), and coral snakes. The first three are pit vipers. The coral snake is small and colorful, with a series of bright red, yellow, and black bands around its body (every other band is yellow). It also has a black snout.

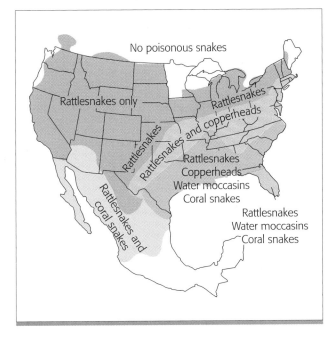

Location of venomous snakes

ANIMAL BITES

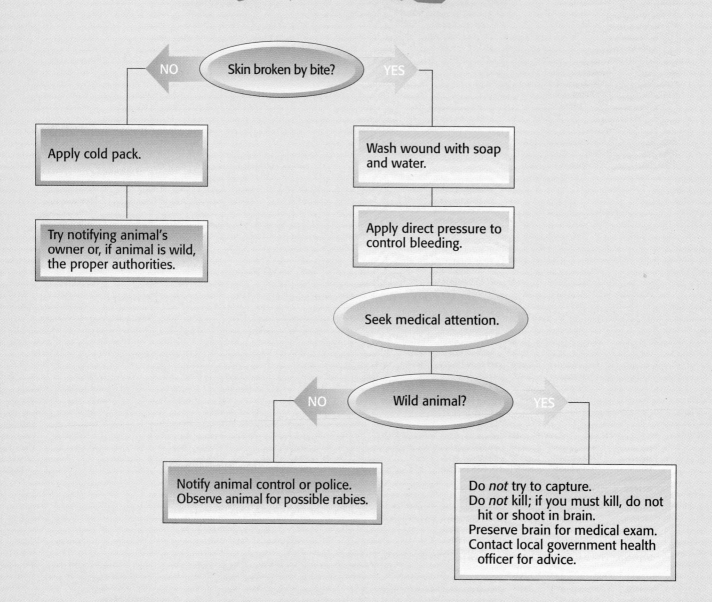

Skin broken by bite?

NO → Apply cold pack.

Try notifying animal's owner or, if animal is wild, the proper authorities.

YES → Wash wound with soap and water.

Apply direct pressure to control bleeding.

Seek medical attention.

Wild animal?

NO → Notify animal control or police. Observe animal for possible rabies.

YES → Do *not* try to capture.
Do *not* kill; if you must kill, do not hit or shoot in brain.
Preserve brain for medical exam.
Contact local government health officer for advice.

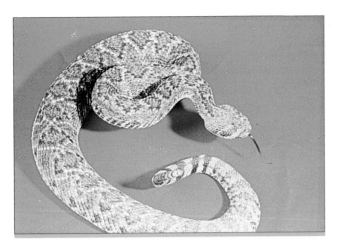

Rattlesnake

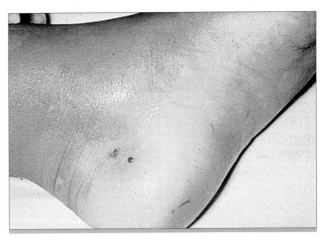

Rattlesnake bite (Note two fang marks)

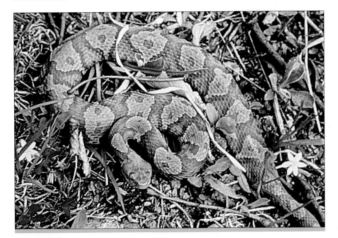

Copperhead snake

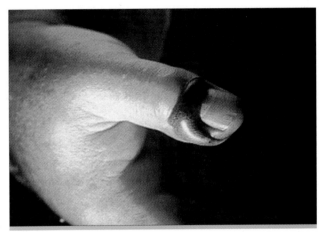

Copperhead bite two hours after bite

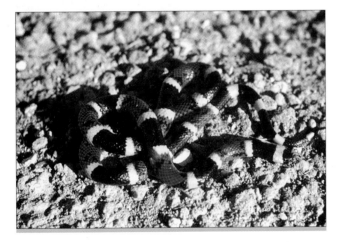

Coral snake, America's most venomous snake

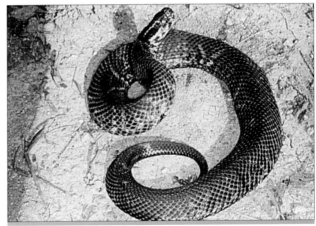

Water moccasin (cottonmouth)

Pit Viper Bites

What to Look For

- severe burning pain at the bite site
- two small puncture wounds about one-half inch apart (some cases may have only one fang mark)
- swelling (happens within 5 minutes and can involve an entire extremity)
- discoloration and blood-filled blisters possibly developing in 6 to 10 hours
- in severe cases, nausea, vomiting, sweating, and weakness

In about 25 percent of poisonous snakebites, there is no venom injection, only fang and tooth wounds (known as a "dry" bite).

What to Do

Identifying the type of pit viper is of minimal importance, since the same antivenin is used to counteract all North American pit viper venom.

The Wilderness Medical Society lists the following guidelines for dealing with bites by pit vipers.

1. Get the victim and bystanders away from the snake. Snakes have been known to bite more than once. Pit vipers can strike about one-half their body length. Be careful around a decapitated snake head—head reactions can persist for 20 minutes or more.
2. Keep the victim quiet. If possible, carry the victim or have the victim walk very slowly to help.
3. Gently wash the bitten area with soap and water.
4. If you are more than one hour from a medical facility with antivenin or if the snake was large and the victim's skin is swelling rapidly, immediately apply suction with the Extractor™ (from Sawyer Products). It does not require cutting.
5. Seek medical attention *immediately*. This is the most important thing to do for the victim.

◤ CAUTION: DO NOT

- apply cold or ice to a snakebite. It does not inactivate the venom and poses a danger of frostbite.
- use the "cut-and-suck" procedure— you could damage underlying structures (e.g., blood vessels, nerves).
- apply mouth suction. Your mouth is filled with bacteria, increasing the likelihood of wound infection.
- apply electric shock.

Coral Snake Bites

The coral snake is America's most venomous snake, but it rarely bites people. The coral snake has short fangs and tends to hang on and "chew" its venom into the victim rather than to strike and release, like a pit viper.

What to Do

1. Keep the victim calm.
2. Gently clean the bite site with soap and water.
3. Apply mild pressure by wrapping several elastic bandages (e.g., Ace™ bandage) over the bite site and the entire arm or leg. Applying such pressure is recommended only for bites from elapid (e.g., coral) snakes, not pit vipers. Do *not* cut the victim's skin or use an Extractor.
4. Seek medical attention for antivenin.

Nonpoisonous Snakebites

A nonpoisonous snake leaves a horseshoe shape of toothmarks on the victim's skin. If you are not positive about a snake, assume it was venomous. Some so-called nonpoisonous North American snakes (e.g., hognose and garter snakes) have venom that can cause painful local reactions but no systemic (whole-body) symptoms.

What to Do

1. Gently clean the bite site with soap and water.
2. Care for the bite as you would a minor wound.
3. Seek medical advice.

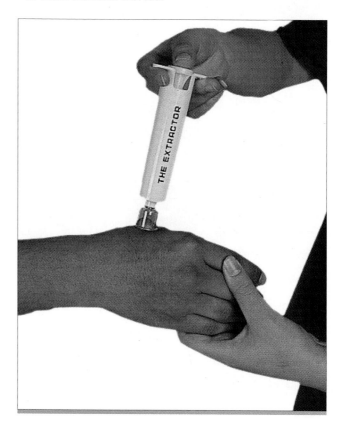

Extractor™ use does not require cutting the skin.

SNAKEBITES

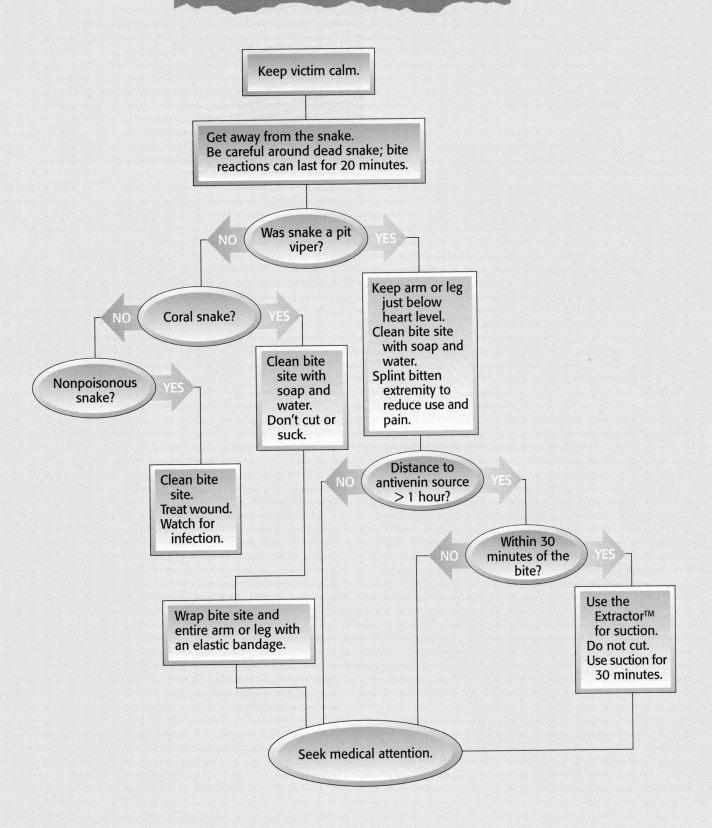

Keep victim calm.

Get away from the snake.
Be careful around dead snake; bite reactions can last for 20 minutes.

Was snake a pit viper?

NO

YES

Coral snake?

NO

YES

Nonpoisonous snake?

NO

YES

Keep arm or leg just below heart level.
Clean bite site with soap and water.
Splint bitten extremity to reduce use and pain.

Clean bite site with soap and water.
Don't cut or suck.

Clean bite site.
Treat wound.
Watch for infection.

Distance to antivenin source > 1 hour?

NO

YES

Within 30 minutes of the bite?

NO

YES

Use the Extractor™ for suction.
Do not cut.
Use suction for 30 minutes.

Wrap bite site and entire arm or leg with an elastic bandage.

Seek medical attention.

Insect Stings

Severe allergic reactions to insect stings are reported by about 0.5 percent of the population in the United States. Fortunately, localized pain, itching, and swelling—the most common consequences of an insect bite—can be treated with first aid.

What to Look For

A rule of thumb is that the sooner symptoms develop after a sting, the more serious the reaction will be.

What to Do

Most people who have been stung can be treated on site, but everyone should know what to do if a life-threatening allergic reaction (anaphylaxis) occurs. In particular, those who have had a severe reaction to an insect sting should be instructed on what they can do to protect themselves. They also should be advised to wear a medical-alert identification tag identifying them as insect allergic.

1. Look at the sting site for a stinger embedded in the skin. Bees are the only stinging insects that leave their stingers behind. If the stinger is still embedded, remove it or it will continue to inject poison for two or three minutes. Scrape the stinger and venom sac away with a hard object such as a long fingernail, credit card, scissor edge, or knife blade. If applied in the first three minutes, a Sawyer Extractor can remove a portion of the venom.

2. Wash the sting site with soap and water to prevent infection.

3. Apply an ice pack over the sting site to slow absorption of the venom and relieve pain. Because bee venom is acidic, a paste made of baking soda and water can help. Sodium bicarbonate is an alkalinizing agent that draws out fluid and reduces itching and swelling.

CAUTION: DO NOT

- pull the stinger with tweezers or your fingers because you may squeeze more venom into the victim from the venom sac.

- use epinephrine unless the victim has a severe allergic reaction.

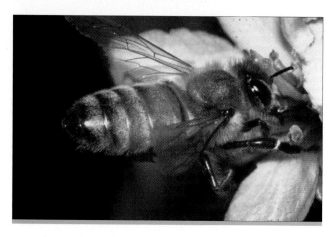

Honeybee

Wasp venom, on the other hand, is alkaline, so apply vinegar or lemon juice.

4. To further relieve pain and itching, some type of analgesic (e.g., aspirin, acetaminophen) usually is adequate. A topical steroid cream, such as hydrocortisone, can help combat local swelling and itching. An antihistamine may prevent some local symptoms if given early, but it works too slowly to counteract a life-threatening allergic reaction.

5. Observe the victim for at least 30 minutes for signs of an allergic reaction. For a person having a severe allergic reaction, a dose of epinephrine is the only effective treatment. A person with a known allergy to insect stings should have a physician-prescribed emergency kit that includes prefilled syringes of epinephrine. Because epinephrine is short-acting, watch the victim closely for signs of returning anaphylaxis. Inject another dose of epinephrine as often as every 15 minutes if needed.

Spider Bites

Most spiders are venomous, which is how they paralyze and kill their prey, but lack an effective delivery system—long fangs and strong jaws to bite a human. Death occurs rarely and only from bites by brown recluse and black widow spiders.

A spider bite is difficult to diagnose, especially when the spider was not seen or recovered, because the bites typically cause little immediate pain.

Black Widow Spiders

Black widow spiders have round abdomens that vary in color from gray to brown to black, depend-

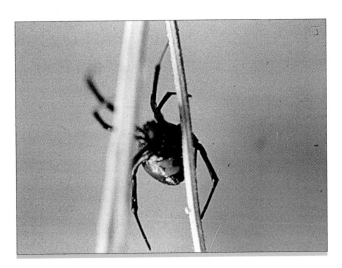

Black widow spider. Note red hourglass configuration on abdomen.

ing on the species. In the female black widow, the abdomen is shiny black with a red or yellow spot (often in the shape of an hourglass) or white spots or bands. Black widow spiders are found throughout the world.

What to Look For

It is difficult to determine if a person has been bitten by a black widow spider or, for that matter, by any spider.

- The victim may feel a sharp pinprick when the spider bites, but some victims are not even aware of the bite. Within 15 minutes, a dull, numbing pain develops in the bite area.
- Two small fang marks might be seen as tiny red spots.
- Within 15 minutes to 4 hours, muscle stiffness and cramps occur, usually affecting the abdomen when the bite is on a lower part of the body and the shoulders, back, or chest when the bite is on an upper part. Victims often describe the pain as the most severe they have ever experienced.
- Headache, chills, fever, heavy sweating, dizziness, nausea, and vomiting appear next. Severe pain around the bite site peaks in 2 to 3 hours and can last 12 to 48 hours.

Brown Recluse Spiders

Brown recluse spiders are also known in North America as fiddle-back, violin, and brown spiders. They have a violin-shaped figure on their backs (several other spider species have a similar configu-

ration on their backs). Color varies from fawn to dark brown, with darker legs.

Brown recluse spiders are found primarily in the southern and midwestern states, with other, less toxic, related spiders throughout the rest of the country. They are absent from the Pacific Northwest.

What to Look For

- A local reaction is usually manifested within two to eight hours by mild to severe pain at the bite site and the development of redness, swelling, and local itching.
- In 48 to 72 hours, a blister develops at the bite site, becomes red, and bursts. During the early stages, the affected area often takes on a bull's-eye appearance, with a central white area surrounded by a reddened area, ringed by a whitish or blue border. A small, red crater remains, over which a scab forms. When that scab falls away in a few days, a still larger crater remains. That too scabs over and falls off, leaving a yet larger crater. The craters are known as *volcano lesions*. This process of slow tissue destruction can continue for weeks or even months. The ulcer sometimes requires skin grafting.
- Fever, weakness, vomiting, joint pain, and a rash may occur.
- Stomach cramps, nausea, and vomiting may occur.

Tarantulas

Tarantulas bite only when vigorously provoked or roughly handled. The bite varies from almost painless to a deep throbbing pain lasting up to one hour. The tarantula, when upset, will roughly scratch the lower surface of its abdomen with its legs and flick hairs onto the invader's skin. The hairs cause itching and hives that can last several weeks. Treatment is cortisone cream and antihistamines.

What to Do (for All Spider Bites)

1. If possible, catch the spider to confirm its identity. Even if the body has been crushed, save it for identification (although most spider-bite victims never see the spider). The species helps determine the treatment, so the dead spider (if it can be found) should be taken with the victim to the hospital.

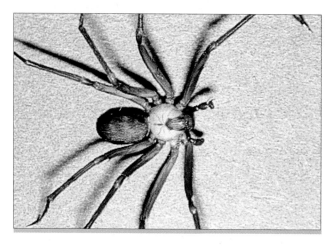

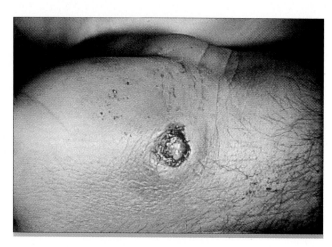

Brown recluse spider. Note violin or fiddle configuration on back.

Brown recluse spider bite. Note bull's-eye approach.

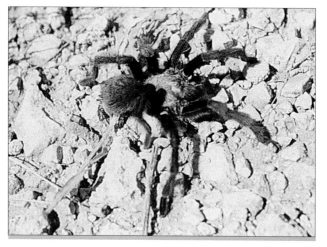

Tarantula

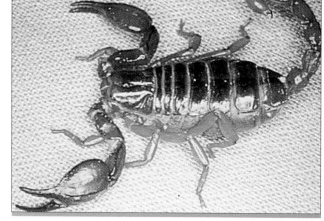

Scorpion

2. Clean the bite area with soap and water or rubbing alcohol.

3. Place an ice pack over the bite to relieve pain and delay the effects of the venom.

4. Monitor the ABCs.

5. Seek medical attention immediately. For black widow spider bites, an antivenin exists. It is usually reserved for children (under 6 years), the elderly (over 60 and with high blood pressure), pregnant women, and victims with severe reactions. The antivenin will give relief within one to three hours. Antivenin for brown recluse and other spider bites is not currently available.

Scorpion Stings

Scorpions look like miniature lobsters, with lobster-like pincers and a long upcurved "tail" with a poisonous stinger. Several species of scorpions inhabit the southwestern United States, but only the bark scorpion poses a threat to humans.

What to Look For

The most frequent symptom of a scorpion sting, especially to an adult victim, is local, immediate pain and burning around the sting site. Later, numbness or tingling occurs.

What to Do

1. Monitor the ABCs.

2. Gently clean the sting site with soap and water or rubbing alcohol.

3. Apply an ice pack over the sting site.

4. Seek medical attention. Small children are prime candidates for receiving antivenin. An antivenin is available only in Arizona.

Mosquito Bites

Millions of people are bitten by mosquitoes. Mosquitoes not only are a nuisance, they also are the carriers of many diseases. In developing countries, mosquitoes transmit malaria, yellow fever, and dengue fever; in the United States, they carry encephalitis. There is no evidence that mosquitoes transmit HIV, the virus that causes AIDS.

What to Do

1. Wash the bitten area with soap and water.
2. Apply an ice pack.
3. Apply calamine lotion to decrease redness and itching.
4. For a victim suffering a number of bites or a delayed allergic reaction, an antihistamine (Benadryl™) every six hours or a physician-prescribed cortisone may prove useful.

Tick Embedded
Removing Ticks

Remove ticks as soon as possible. If a tick is carrying a disease, the longer it stays embedded, the greater the chance of the disease being transmitted.

Because its bite is painless, a tick can remain embedded for days without the victim realizing it. Most tick bites are harmless, although ticks can carry serious diseases.

1. To pull a tick off,
   - Use tweezers if possible. If you have to use your fingers, protect your skin by using a paper towel or disposable tissue or gloves.
   - Grasp the tick as close to the skin surface as possible and pull away from the skin with a steady pressure. Or lift the tick slightly upward and pull parallel to the skin until the tick detaches.
2. Wash the bite site with soap and water. Apply rubbing alcohol to further disinfect the area.

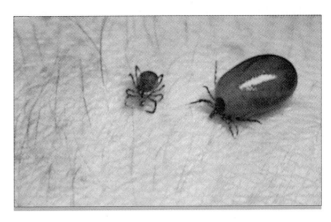

Deer ticks: not engorged and blood engorged

 CAUTION: DO NOT

- use the following popular methods of tick removal, which have been proved useless:
  - petroleum jelly
  - fingernail polish
  - rubbing alcohol
  - a hot match
  - a petroleum product, such as gasoline
- grab a tick at the rear of its body. The internal gut may rupture and the contents be squeezed out, causing infection.
- twist or jerk the tick, which may result in incomplete removal.

3. Apply an ice pack to reduce pain.
4. Apply calamine lotion to relieve any itching. Keep the area clean.
5. Continue to watch the bite site for one month for a rash. If a rash appears, see a physician. Watch for other signs such as fever, muscle aches, sensitivity to bright light, and paralysis that begins with leg weakness.

Bites and Stings

Directions: Circle Yes if you agree with the statement, and circle No if you disagree.

Yes   No   1. Report animal bites to the police or animal control officers.

Yes   No   2. Apply cold or ice over a snakebite.

Yes   No   3. Use the "cut-and-suck" method for a snakebite.

Yes   No   4. In remote settings, suction snake venom out with an Extractor.

Yes   No   5. Apply a cold or ice pack over an insect sting or a suspected spider bite.

Yes   No   6. A baking soda paste can help reduce itching and swelling caused by an insect sting.

Yes   No   7. A victim's doctor-prescribed epinephrine may have to be given if the victim has a life-threatening reaction to an insect sting.

Yes   No   8. Spider bite antivenin is available for only black widow spider bites, and not all victims need it.

Yes   No   9. An antihistamine or cortisone can be useful for mosquito bites.

Yes   No   10. Apply a blown-out, glowing match head or heated needle to cause an embedded tick to back out of a victim's skin.

Yes   No   11. Cover an embedded tick with heavy oil or grease to cause a tick to back out because of lack of oxygen.

Scenario #1: A mail carrier is heard crying for help while being attacked by a neighbor's large dog. The dog's owner calls off the dog and takes it inside his house. You run up the street and help the victim over to a nearby yard. You find several severe bite marks on the mail carrier's legs and arms. What should you do?

_____

_____

Scenario #2: You rush to a vacant lot to help a young woman who is calling for help. She says that some type of snake bit her on the leg. You see two puncture wounds (fang marks) on her leg. What should you do?

_____

_____

Scenario #3: A garden shop employee complains about her face swelling and a feeling of tightness across her chest. She is having some breathing difficulty. She says a bee stung her. She has a medical alert tag around her neck indicating an allergy to insects. She tells you that she has medication for such an emergency. There is an ice machine nearby. What should you do?

_____

_____

Scenario #4: While resting during lunch in a company office patio, you feel a sharp pinprick on your arm. About 15 minutes later, dull, numbing pain develops in your back. You look at your arm and see two tiny red spots. About an hour later, abdominal cramping starts and steadily gets worse. What should you do?

_____

_____

Scenario #5: On a Monday morning, one of your co-workers returns from a weekend camping trip. When he rubs the back of his head, he feels a bump and asks you to look at it. You see a tick embedded in his scalp. What should you do?

_____

_____

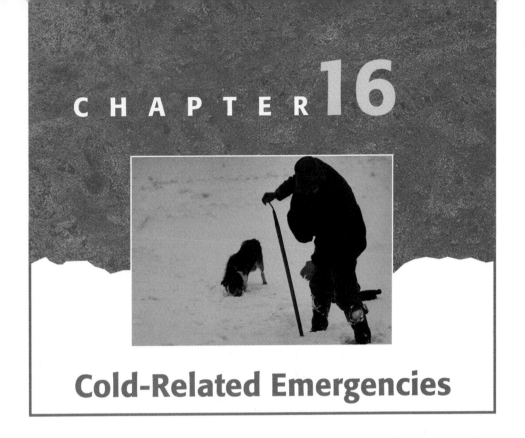

CHAPTER 16

Cold-Related Emergencies

Freezing Cold Injuries

Freezing cold injuries can occur whenever the air temperature is below freezing (32°F). Freezing limited to the skin surface is frostnip. Freezing that extends deeper through the skin and into the flesh is frostbite.

Frostnip involves the freezing of water on the skin surface. The skin becomes reddened and possibly swollen. Although painful, there usually is no further damage after rewarming. Repeated frostnip in the same spot can dry the skin, causing it to crack and become sensitive. It is difficult to tell the difference between frostnip and frostbite. Frostnip should be taken seriously since it may be the first sign of impending frostbite. First aid for frostnip consists of gently warming the affected area by placing it against a warm body part (e.g., bare hands, armpit, stomach) or by blowing warm air on the area. Do not rub the area. After rewarming, the affected area may be red and tingling.

Frostbite occurs when temperatures drop below freezing. Frostbite affects mainly the feet, hands, ears, and nose. Those areas do not contain large heat-producing muscles and are some distance from the body's heat-generation sources. The most severe consequences of frostbite are gangrene and amputation.

What to Look For

The severity and extent of frostbite are difficult to judge until hours after thawing, although before thawing it can be classified as *superficial* or *deep*. Even physicians have to wait until thawing has occurred before they can judge the extent of the injury.

The signs and symptoms of superficial frostbite are as follows:

- Skin color is white, waxy, or grayish-yellow.

- The affected part feels very cold and numb. There may be tingling, stinging, or an aching sensation.
- The skin surface feels stiff or crusty and the underlying tissue soft when depressed gently and firmly.

Deep frostbite is indicated by the following signs and symptoms:

- The affected part feels cold, hard, and solid and cannot be depressed.
- The affected part is cold, with pale, waxy skin.
- A painfully cold part suddenly stops hurting.
- Blisters may appear after rewarming.

After a part has thawed, frostbite can be categorized by degrees, similar to the classification of burns.

What to Do

All frostbite injuries require the same first aid treatment.

1. Get the victim out of the cold and to a warm place.
2. Remove any clothing or constricting items that could impair blood circulation (e.g., rings).
3. Seek immediate medical attention.
4. If the affected part is partially thawed or the victim is in a remote or wilderness situation (more than 1 hour from a medical facility), use the following wet, rapid rewarming method.
   Place the frostbitten part in warm (102°–105°F) water. If you do not have a thermometer, pour some of the water over the

Table 16.1: How Cold Is It?

In addition to coldness, two other factors account for body heat loss: moisture and wind. Moisture—whether from rain, snow, or perspiration—speeds the conduction of heat away from the body.

Wind causes sizable amounts of body-heat loss. If the thermometer reads 20°F and the wind speed is 20 mph, the exposure is comparable to −10°F. This is called the windchill factor. Use the following rough measures of wind speed: If you feel the wind on your face, the speed is about 10 mph; if small branches move or dust or snow is raised,

20 mph; if large branches are moving, 30 mph; and if a whole tree bends, about 40 mph.

To determine the windchill factor:

1. Estimate the wind speed by checking for the signs described above.
2. Look at a thermometer reading (in Fahrenheit degrees) outdoors.
3. Match the estimated wind speed with the actual thermometer reading in the table below.

Windchill Factor

Estimated Wind Speed (mph)	Actual Thermometer Reading (°F)											
	50	40	30	20	10	0	−10	−20	−30	−40	−50	−60
	Equivalent Temperature (°F)											
Calm	50	40	30	20	10	0	−10	−20	−30	−40	−50	−60
5	48	37	27	16	6	−5	−15	−26	−36	−47	−57	−68
10	40	28	16	3	−9	−21	−33	−46	−58	−70	−83	−95
15	36	22	9	−5	−18	−32	−45	−58	−72	−85	−99	−112
20	32	18	4	−10	−25	−39	−53	−67	−82	−96	−110	−124
25	30	15	0	−15	−29	−44	−59	−74	−89	−104	−118	−133
30	25	13	−2	−18	−33	−48	−63	−79	−94	−109	−125	−140
35	27	11	−4	−20	−35	−51	−67	−82	−98	−113	−129	−145
40	26	10	−6	−21	−37	−53	−69	−85	−101	−117	−132	−148

(Wind speeds greater than 40 mph have little additional effect.)

Little danger. (In less than 5 hours with dry skin. Greatest hazard from false sense of security.)

Increasing danger. (Exposed flesh may freeze within 1 minute.)

Great danger. (Flesh may freeze within 30 seconds.)

⚠ CAUTION: DO NOT

- rub or massage the part—ice crystals can be pushed into body cells, rupturing them.
- rewarm the part with a heating pad, hot-water bottle, stove, sunlamp, radiator, or exhaust pipe or over a fire. Excessive temperatures cannot be controlled, resulting in burns.
- allow the victim to drink alcoholic beverages. Alcohol dilates blood vessels and causes a loss of body heat.
- allow the victim to smoke. Smoking constricts blood vessels, thus impairing circulation.
- rewarm if there is any possibility of refreezing.
- allow the thawed part to refreeze since ice crystals formed will be larger and more damaging. If refreezing is likely or even possible, it is better to leave the part frozen.
- use the "dry" rewarming technique (putting the victim's hands in your armpits) since that takes three to four times longer than the wet, rapid method to thaw frozen tissue. Slow rewarming results in greater tissue damage than rapid rewarming.

....

inside of your arm or put your elbow into it to test that it is warm, not hot. Maintain water temperature by adding warm water. Rewarming usually takes 20 to 40 minutes or until the tissues are soft. To help control the severe pain

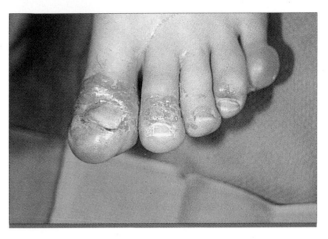

Second-degree frostbite

during rewarming, give the victim aspirin or ibuprofen. For ear or facial injuries, apply warm moist cloths, changing them frequently.

5. After thawing,
- Treat victim as a "stretcher" case—the feet will be impossible to use after they are rewarmed.
- Protect the affected area from contact with clothing and bedding.
- Place dry, sterile gauze between the toes and the fingers to absorb moisture and to keep them from sticking together.

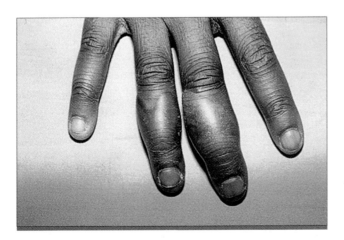

Frostbitten fingers, 6 hours after rewarming in 108°F water

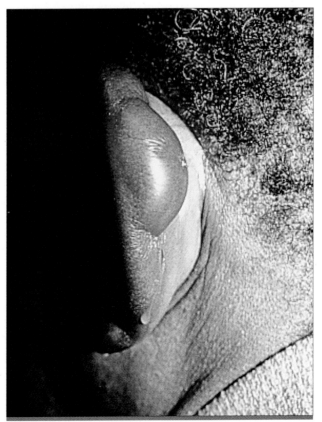

Frostbitten ear 8 hours old

FROSTBITE

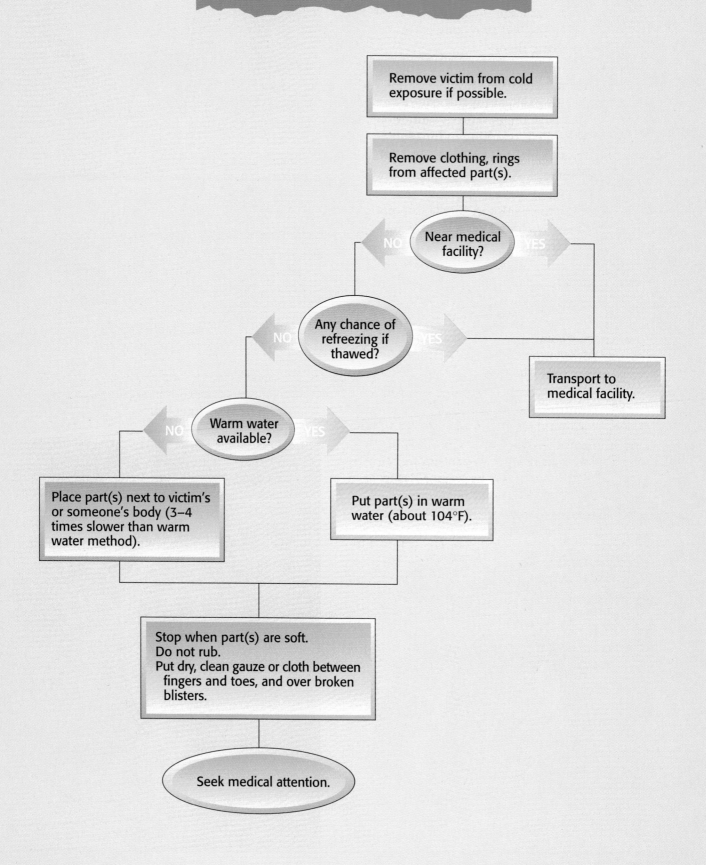

Remove victim from cold exposure if possible.

Remove clothing, rings from affected part(s).

Near medical facility?

NO → YES → Transport to medical facility.

Any chance of refreezing if thawed?

NO → YES

Warm water available?

NO → Place part(s) next to victim's or someone's body (3–4 times slower than warm water method).

YES → Put part(s) in warm water (about 104°F).

Stop when part(s) are soft.
Do not rub.
Put dry, clean gauze or cloth between fingers and toes, and over broken blisters.

Seek medical attention.

- Slightly elevate the affected part to reduce pain and swelling.
- Apply aloe vera gel to promote skin healing.
- Give the victim aspirin or ibuprofen to limit pain and inflammation.

Hypothermia

Body temperature falls when the body cannot produce heat as fast as it is being lost. Hypothermia is a life-threatening condition when the body's core temperature falls below 95°F.

It can happen indoors, in the southern states, and even on a summer day. It does not require subfreezing temperatures.

What to Look For

- *Change in mental status.* Deteriorated responsiveness or mental status is one of the first symptoms of developing hypothermia. Examples are disorientation, apathy, and changes in personality, such as unusual aggressiveness.
- *Shivering.* Shivering is the first, and most important, body defense against a falling body temperature. *Shivering* starts when the body temperature drops 1°F and *can produce more heat than many rewarming methods.* As the core temperature continues to fall, shivering usually stops at about 90°F. Shivering also stops as body temperature rises. If shivering stops while responsiveness is decreasing, assume that the core temperature is falling. If, on the other hand, shivering stops while the victim is becoming more coordinated and feeling better, assume that the core temperature is rising.
- *Cool abdomen.* Place the back of your hand between the clothing and the victim's abdomen to assess the victim's temperature. When the victim's abdominal skin under clothing is cooler than your hand, consider the victim hypothermic until proved otherwise.
- *Low core body temperature.* The best indicator of hypothermia is a thermometer reading of the core body temperature. Normal thermometers do not register below 94°F and so do not indicate whether the hypothermia is mild or severe. Because first aid for mild hypothermia is different from that for severe hypothermia, it is helpful to have a thermometer that registers below 90°F. However, measuring rectal temperatures is seldom done, mainly because low-reading rectal thermometers usually are not readily available. Also, taking a rectal temperature can be difficult, inconvenient, and embarrassing to victim and rescuer. If done outdoors, such a procedure can expose the already cold victim.

Types of Hypothermia

The difference between mild and severe hypothermia is based on the core body temperature, but taking a rectal temperature often is not possible. The other most significant difference is that with severe hypothermia the victim becomes so cold that shivering stops. That means the victim's body cannot rewarm itself internally and will require external heat for recovery.

Victims of mild hypothermia have a core body temperature above 90°F. Symptoms are shivering, slurred speech, memory lapses, and fumbling hands. Victims frequently stumble and stagger, but they are usually responsive and can talk. While many people suffer cold hands and feet, victims of mild hypothermia experience cold abdomens.

Victims of severe hypothermia have a core body temperature below 90°F. Shivering has stopped. Muscles may be stiff and rigid, similar to rigor mortis. The victim's skin is ice cold and has a blue appearance. Pulse and breathing slow down, and the pupils dilate. The victim appears to be dead.

What to Do

1. For all hypothermic victims, stop further heat loss:
   - Get the victim out of the cold.
   - Handle the victim gently. Rough handling can cause a cardiac arrest.
   - Replace wet clothing with dry clothing.
   - Add insulation (e.g., blankets, towels, pillows, newspapers) beneath and around the victim. Cover the victim's head (50–80 percent of the body's heat loss is through the head).
   - Keep the victim in a horizontal (flat) position.
2. Call the EMS for immediate medical transportation. Remember that hypothermia is more common in urban settings than in victims found in the wilderness.
3. For mild hypothermia in a remote or wilderness location, the goal is to prevent further heat loss. If protected from further heat loss, most mildly hypothermic victims are able to rewarm themselves by shivering, which generates heat.

HYPOTHERMIA

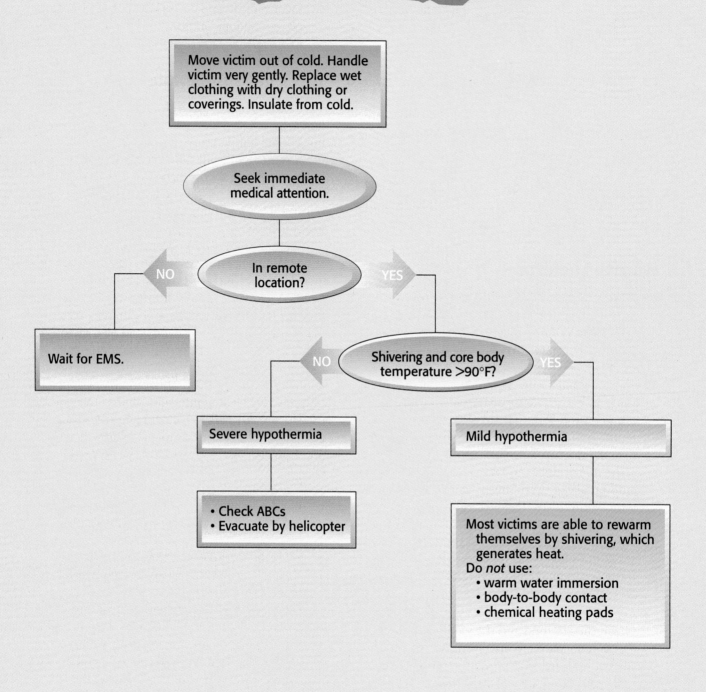

Move victim out of cold. Handle victim very gently. Replace wet clothing with dry clothing or coverings. Insulate from cold.

Seek immediate medical attention.

In remote location?

NO → Wait for EMS.

YES → Shivering and core body temperature >90°F?

NO → Severe hypothermia
- Check ABCs
- Evacuate by helicopter

YES → Mild hypothermia

Most victims are able to rewarm themselves by shivering, which generates heat.
Do *not* use:
- warm water immersion
- body-to-body contact
- chemical heating pads

4. For severe hypothermia in a remote or wilderness situation:
   - Check the victim's ABCs (airway, breathing, circulation). Take 30 to 45 seconds to check the pulse before starting CPR.
   - Evacuate the victim by helicopter. Rewarming in a remote location is difficult and rarely effective.

Adding heat to a victim is extremely difficult. The longer the victim has been exposed to the cold, the longer it will take to raise the core temperature to normal. Trying to rewarm a hypothermic victim may cause a cardiac arrest.

Although surface rewarming suppresses shivering, it may be the only option when the victim is far from medical care. In that case, the victim must be warmed by any available external heat source.

Frostbite

Directions: Circle Yes if you agree with the statement, and circle No if you disagree.

Yes   No   1. Rub or massage to rewarm a frostbitten part.

Yes   No   2. Frostbite damage becomes more severe if the affected area is thawed and then refrozen.

Yes   No   3. It's best to rewarm a frostbitten part by using warm water.

Yes   No   4. Placing frostbitten hands in another person's armpits is the best rewarming method.

Yes   No   5. When near a hospital, it's best to let medical personnel thaw the frostbitten part.

Scenario: In subfreezing temperatures and during a snowstorm, you find a stalled truck on a little-used road. Inside the truck is an elderly man, who tells you that his truck is out of gasoline and that when he tried to refill the truck's gas tank he dropped the gas can with some of the gasoline spilling on his hands. He has been stranded for over 3 hours. The man complains of numb fingers and cold feet. He did not know about a cabin about a quarter mile away. What should you do?

_____

_____

_____

Hypothermia

Yes   No   1. Add insulation (blankets) around and under the victim.

Yes   No   2. Replace wet clothing with dry clothing.

Yes   No   3. Shivering is sufficient to rewarm a mild hypothermic victim.

Yes   No   4. For mild hypothermia, applying chemical heat packs or using a rescuer's body heat are preferred methods of rewarming a victim.

Yes   No   5. Severe hypothermic victims should be transported to a hospital for rewarming.

Yes   No   6. Check a severe hypothermic victim's pulse for at least 30 to 45 seconds.

Scenario: It is a cold winter day so you decide to check on your 80-year-old grandfather, who lives alone. As you enter his home, you notice that it is not much warmer inside the house than it is outside. You find your grandfather wrapped in a blanket lying on top of his bed. You speak to him, but you get only mumbling. He is severely shivering. What should you do?

_____

_____

_____

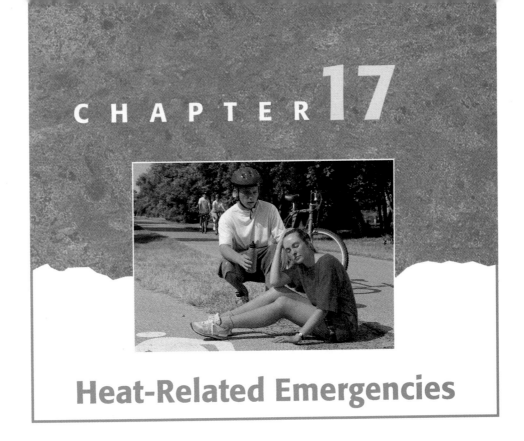

CHAPTER 17

Heat-Related Emergencies

Heat Illnesses

Several disorders exist along a spectrum of heat illnesses. Some of them are common, but only heatstroke is life threatening. Untreated heatstroke victims always die.

Heat Cramps

Heat cramps are painful muscular spasms that happen suddenly. They usually involve the back of the leg muscles (calf and hamstring muscles) or the abdominal muscles. They tend to happen immediately after exertion and some experts claim they are caused by salt depletion. Victims may be drinking water without adequate salt content. However, some experts disagree because the typical American diet is heavy with salt.

Heat Exhaustion

Heat exhaustion is characterized by heavy perspiration with normal or slightly above normal body temperatures. It is caused by water or salt depletion or both. Some experts believe that a better term would be severe dehydration. Heat exhaustion affects workers and athletes who do not drink enough fluids while working or exercising in hot environments. Symptoms include severe thirst, fatigue, headache, nausea, vomiting, and sometimes diarrhea. The affected person often mistakenly believes he or she has the flu. Uncontrolled heat exhaustion can evolve into heatstroke.

Heatstroke

Two types of heatstroke exist: classic and exertional. Classic heatstroke, also known as the "slow cooker," may take days to develop. It is often seen during summer heat waves and typically affects poor, elderly, chronically ill, alcoholic, or obese persons. Because the elderly, often with medical problems, are frequently afflicted, this type of heatstroke has a 50-percent death rate even with medical care. It results from a combination of a hot environment and dehydration. Exertional heatstroke is also more common in the summer. It is frequently seen in athletes, laborers, and military personnel, all of whom often sweat profusely. This type of heatstroke is known as the "fast cooker." It affects healthy, active individuals strenuously working or playing in a warm environment. Because its rapid onset does not allow enough time for severe dehydration to occur, 50 percent of exertional heatstroke victims usually are sweating. (Classic heatstroke victims are not sweating.)

There are several ways to tell the difference between heat exhaustion and heatstroke. First, if the victim's body feels extremely hot when touched, suspect heatstroke. Another major mark of heatstroke is altered mental status (behavior), ranging from slight confusion and disorientation to coma. Between those extreme conditions, victims usually become irrational, agitated, or even aggressive and may have seizures. In severe cases, the victim can go into a coma in less than an hour. The longer a coma lasts, the less the chance for survival.

A third way to distinguish heatstroke from heat exhaustion is by rectal temperature. That is not very practical, however, because a responsive heatstroke victim may not cooperate. Taking a rectal temperature can be embarrassing to both victim and rescuer. Moreover, rectal thermometers are seldom available.

Other Heat Illnesses

Less serious heat illnesses include heat syncope, heat edema, and prickly heat:

- Heat syncope, in which a person becomes dizzy or faints after exposure to high temperatures, is a self-limiting condition. Victims should lie down in a cool place and, if not nauseated, drink water.

- Heat edema, which is also a self-limiting condition, causes the ankles and feet to swell from heat exposure. It is more common in women unacclimatized to a hot climate. It is related to salt and water retention and tends to disappear after acclimatization. Wearing support stockings and elevating the legs may help reduce the swelling.

- Prickly heat, also known as a heat rash, is an itchy rash that develops because of unevaporated moisture on skin wet from sweating. Treat by drying and cooling the skin.

What to Do

Heat Cramps
To relieve heat cramps (it may take several hours), follow these steps:

1. Rest in a cool place.
2. Drink lightly salted cool water (dissolve ¼ teaspoon salt in a quart of water) or a commercial sports drink.
3. Stretch the cramped calf muscle. Also, try an acupressure method: pinch the upper lip just below the nose.

Heat Exhaustion

1. Move the victim immediately out of the heat to a cool place.
2. Give cool liquids, adding electrolytes (lightly salted water or a commercial sports drink) if plain water does not improve the victim's condition in 20 minutes. Do not give salt tablets; they can irritate the stomach and cause nausea and vomiting.
3. Raise the victim's legs 8 to 12 inches (keep the legs straight).
4. Remove excess clothing.
5. Sponge with cool water and fan the victim.
6. If no improvement is seen within 30 minutes, seek medical attention.

Heatstroke
Heatstroke is a medical emergency and must be treated rapidly! Every minute delayed increases the likelihood of serious complications or death.

1. Move the victim immediately out of the heat to a cool place.
2. Remove clothing down to the victim's underwear.
3. Keep the victim's head and shoulders slightly elevated.
4. Seek immediate medical attention, even if the victim seems to be recovering.
5. The only way to prevent damage is to cool the victim quickly and by any means possible. Cooling methods include the following:
   - *Spraying* the victim with water and then *fanning* him or her is another method for cooling

the body. The water droplets act as artificial sweat and cool through evaporation. This method is effective in low-humidity (less than 75 percent) conditions.

- *Ice bags* wrapped in wet towels and placed against the large veins in the groin, armpits, and sides of the neck cool the body in high-humidity (greater than 75 percent) conditions.

CAUTION: DO NOT

- delay initiating cooling while waiting for an ambulance. The longer the delay, the greater the risk of tissue damage and prolonged hospitalization.
- continue cooling after the victim's mental status has improved. Unnecessary cooling could lead to hypothermia.
- use rubbing alcohol to cool the skin. It can be absorbed into the blood and cause alcohol poisoning. Also, the vapors are a potential fire hazard.

How Hot It Feels

Under normal conditions, temperature and humidity are the most important elements influencing body comfort. The Heat Index compiled by the National Weather Service lists apparent temperatures—how hot it feels—at various combinations of temperature and humidity.

Table 17-1: Heat Index

Relative Humidity, %	Air Temperature, °F										
	70	75	80	85	90	95	100	105	110	115	120
	Apparent Temperature, °F										
0	64	69	73	78	83	87	91	95	99	103	107
10	65	70	75	80	85	90	95	100	105	111	116
20	66	72	77	82	87	93	99	105	112	120	130
30	67	73	78	84	90	96	104	113	123	135	148
40	68	74	79	86	93	101	110	123	137	151	
50	69	75	81	88	96	107	120	135	150		
60	70	76	82	90	100	114	132	149			
70	70	77	85	93	106	124	144				
80	71	78	86	97	113	136					
90	71	79	88	102	122						
100	72	80	91	108							

Above 130°F = heatstroke imminent
105°–130°F = heat exhaustion and heat cramps likely; heatstroke with long exposure and activity
90°–105°F = heat exhaustion and heat cramps with long exposure and activity
80°–90°F = fatigue during exposure and activity

Source: National Weather Service.

HEAT-RELATED EMERGENCIES

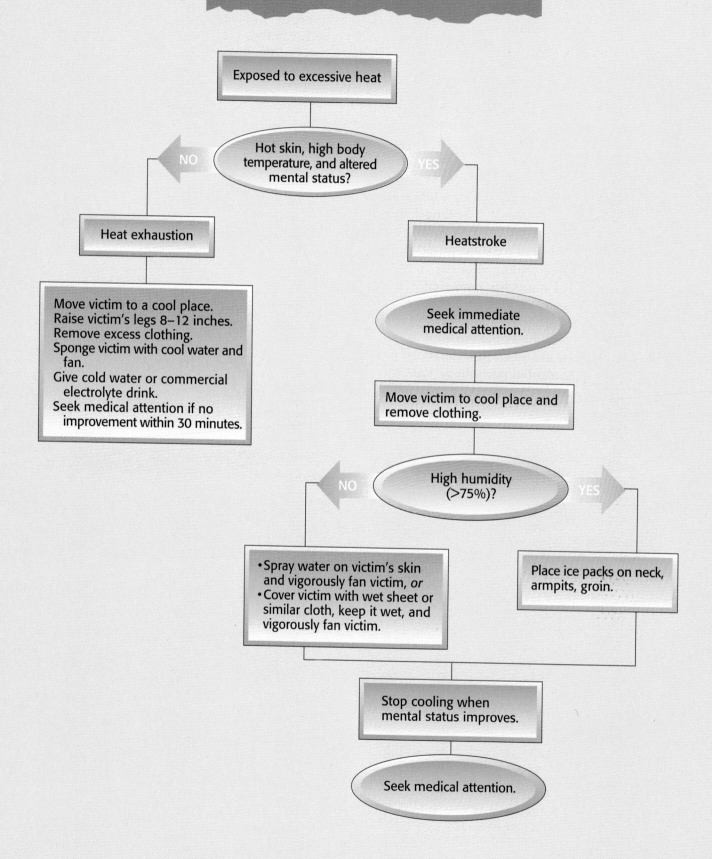

Exposed to excessive heat

Hot skin, high body temperature, and altered mental status?

NO → Heat exhaustion

Move victim to a cool place.
Raise victim's legs 8–12 inches.
Remove excess clothing.
Sponge victim with cool water and fan.
Give cold water or commercial electrolyte drink.
Seek medical attention if no improvement within 30 minutes.

YES → Heatstroke

Seek immediate medical attention.

Move victim to cool place and remove clothing.

High humidity (>75%)?

NO →
• Spray water on victim's skin and vigorously fan victim, *or*
• Cover victim with wet sheet or similar cloth, keep it wet, and vigorously fan victim.

YES → Place ice packs on neck, armpits, groin.

Stop cooling when mental status improves.

Seek medical attention.

LEARNING ACTIVITIES 17

Heat-Related Emergencies

Directions: Circle Yes if you agree with the statement, and circle No if you disagree.

Yes   No   1. For heat cramps, stretch a cramped leg muscle.

Yes   No   2. Salt tablets can be given to victims of any heat illness.

Yes   No   3. Move heat illness victims out of the heat to a cool place.

Yes   No   4. Heat exhaustion victims need immediate medical attention—it's a life-threatening condition.

Yes   No   5. Heatstroke victims need immediate cooling by any means possible.

Yes   No   6. Apply rubbing alcohol on a heatstroke victim's skin for cooling.

Yes   No   7. If in high humid conditions, wet down or spray and fan the heatstroke victim.

Yes   No   8. If in low humid conditions, only cold or ice packs applied to the neck, armpits, and groin will work well to cool a heatstroke victim.

Scenario #1: A teenager's summer job is mowing lawns for various companies in an industrial park. He is sweating heavily on a very hot, humid day. He complains about being very thirsty, nauseous, and having a headache. What should you do?

_____

_____

_____

Scenario #2: On your vacation, you spend a day at a large amusement park. It is an extremely hot and humid day. During the afternoon, you decide to rest and watch one of the special shows. Soon after you have been seated, an elderly man in front of you suddenly falls forward out of his seat. When you reach him, his wife reports that they have been walking around the park practically all day without stopping. His skin feels very hot and dry, and he is unresponsive. What should you do?

_____

_____

_____

Scenario #3: A high-ranking company official from Buffalo has flown to Florida to inspect a new assembly plant. He is accustomed to the cold conditions of the north but not to the heat and humidity of the southeast. He has spent the morning inspecting the new plant. Satisfied with what he's seen, he accepts an invitation to golf in the afternoon. While putting at the sixteenth hole, he becomes dizzy and faints but soon becomes responsive. What should you do?

_____

_____

_____

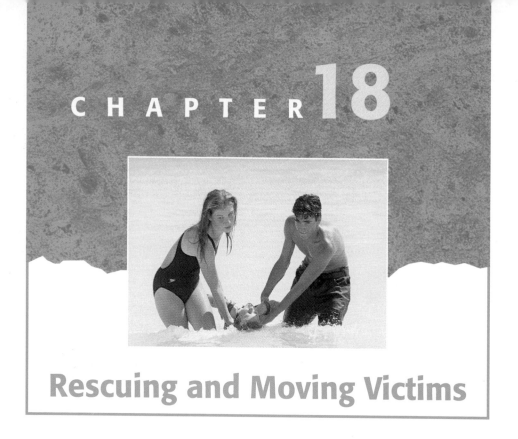

CHAPTER 18

Rescuing and Moving Victims

Victim Rescue

Water Rescue

Reach-throw-row-go identifies the sequence for attempting a water rescue. The first and simplest rescue technique is to *reach* for the victim. Reaching requires a lightweight pole, ladder, long stick, or any object that can be extended to the victim. Once you have your "reacher," secure your footing and have a bystander grab your belt or pants for stability. Secure yourself before reaching for the victim.

You can *throw* anything that floats—empty picnic jug, empty fuel or paint can, life jacket, floating cushion, piece of wood, inflated spare wheel—whatever is available. If there is a rope handy, tie it to the object to be thrown so you can pull the victim in, or, if you miss, you can retrieve the object and throw it again. The average untrained rescuer has a throwing range of about 50 feet.

If the victim is out of throwing range and there is a rowboat, canoe, motor boat, or boogie board nearby, you can try to *row* to the victim. Maneuvering these craft requires skill learned through practice. Wear a personal flotation device (PFD) for your own safety. To avoid capsizing, never pull the victim in over the side of a boat but over the stern (rear end).

If the three techniques are impossible and you are a capable swimmer trained in water lifesaving procedures, you can *go* to the drowning victim by swimming. Entering even calm water to make a swimming rescue is difficult and hazardous. All too often a would-be rescuer becomes a victim as well.

CAUTION: DO NOT

- swim to and grasp a drowning person unless you are trained in lifesaving.

Ice Rescue

If a person has fallen through the ice near the shore, extend a pole or throw a line with a floatable object attached to it. When the person has a hold, pull him or her toward the shore or the edge of the ice.

If the person is through the ice away from the shore and you cannot reach him or her with a pole or a throwing line, lie flat and push a ladder, plank, or similar object ahead of you. If you have nothing but a spare wheel, tie a rope to the wheel and the other end to an anchor point, lie flat, and push the wheel ahead of you. Pull the person ashore or to the edge of the ice.

CAUTION: DO NOT

- go near broken ice without support.

Electrical Emergency Rescue

Electrical injuries are devastating. Even just a mild shock can cause serious internal injuries. A current of 1,000 volts or more is considered high voltage, but even the 110 volts of household current can be deadly.

When a person gets an electric shock, electricity enters the body at the point of contact and travels along the path of least resistance (nerves and blood vessels). The current travels rapidly, generating heat and causing destruction.

Most indoor electrocutions are caused by faulty electrical equipment or careless use of electrical appliances. Before you touch the victim, turn off the

CAUTION: DO NOT

- touch an appliance or the victim until the current is off.
- try to move downed wires.
- use *any* object, even dry wood (e.g., broomstick, tools, chair, stool) to separate the victim from the electrical source.

electricity at the circuit breaker, fuse box, or outside switch box or unplug the appliance if the plug is undamaged.

If the electrocution involves high-voltage *power lines,* the power must be turned off before anyone approaches a victim. If you approach a victim and feel a tingling sensation in your legs and lower body, stop. You are on energized ground, and an electrical current is entering one foot, passing through your lower body, then leaving through the other foot. If that happens, raise one foot off the ground, turn around, and hop to a safe place. Wait for trained personnel with the proper equipment to cut the wires or disconnect them.

If a power line has fallen over a car, tell the driver and passengers to stay in the car. A victim should try to jump out of the car *only* if an explosion or fire threatens, and then without making contact with the car or the wire.

Hazardous Materials Incidents

At almost any highway accident scene, there is the potential danger of hazardous chemicals. Clues that indicate the presence of hazardous materials include

- signs on vehicles (e.g., "explosive," "flammable," "corrosive")
- spilled liquids or solids
- strong, unusual odors
- clouds of vapor

Stay well away and upwind from the area. Only persons who are specially trained in handling hazardous materials and who have the proper equipment should be in the area.

Motor Vehicle Accidents

In most states, you are legally obligated to stop and give help when you are involved in a motor vehicle accident. If you come on an accident shortly after it happens, the law does not require you to stop, although it might be argued that you have a moral responsibility to render any aid you can.

1. Stop your vehicle in a safe place. If the police have taken charge, do not stop unless you are asked to do so.
2. Turn on your flashing hazard lights.
3. Direct bystanders to warn other drivers and to set up warning flares.

4. Try to enter an involved vehicle through a door. If the doors are jammed, try to get someone inside the car to roll down a window. As a last resort, break a window to gain access. Once inside, place the vehicle in park, turn off the key, and set the parking brake.

CAUTION: DO NOT

- rush to get victims out of a car that has been in an accident. Contrary to opinion, most vehicle crashes do not involve fire, and most vehicles stay in an upright position.

5. For unresponsive victims and those who might have spine injuries, use your hands to stabilize their heads and necks.
6. Treat any life-threatening injuries.
7. Whenever possible, wait for EMS personnel to extricate the victims because of their training and having the proper equipment. In most cases, keep the victims stabilized inside the vehicle.

Fires

Should you encounter a fire, you should

1. Get all the people out fast.
2. Call the emergency telephone number (usually 911).

Then—and *only* then—if the fire is small and if your own escape route is clear should you fight the fire yourself with a fire extinguisher. You may be able to put out the fire or at least hold damage to a minimum.

If clothing catches fire, tear it off away from the face. Keep the victim from running, since that fans the flames. Wrap a rug or a woolen blanket around the victim's neck to keep the fire from the face or throw a blanket on the victim. In some cases, you may be able to smother the flames by throwing the victim to the floor and rolling him or her in a rug.

CAUTION: DO NOT

- let a victim run if clothing is on fire.
- get trapped while fighting a fire. Always keep a door behind you so you can exit if the fire gets too big.

To use a fire extinguisher, aim directly at whatever is burning and sweep across it. Extinguishers expel their contents quickly, in 8 to 25 seconds for most home models containing dry chemicals.

Confined Spaces

A confined space is any area not intended for human occupancy that also has the potential for containing or accumulating a dangerous atmosphere. Examples of confined spaces are tanks, vessels, vats, bins, vaults, trenches, and pits.

An accident in a confined space demands immediate action. If an entrant into a confined space signals for help or becomes unconscious, follow these steps to help:

1. Call for immediate help.
2. Do *not* rush in to help.
3. If you are the attendant, do *not* enter the confined space unless you are relieved by another attendant *and* you are part of the rescue team.
4. When help arrives, try to rescue the victim without entering the space.
5. If rescue from the outside cannot be done, allow trained and properly equipped (respiratory protection plus safety harnesses or lifelines) rescuers to enter the space and remove the victim.
6. Activate the local EMS.
7. Give first aid, rescue breathing, or CPR if necessary and if you are trained.

Triage: What to Do with Multiple Victims

You may encounter emergency situations in which there are two or more victims. This often is the case in multiple-car accidents or disasters. After making a quick scene survey, decide who must be cared for and transported first. This process of prioritizing or classifying injured victims is called triage. *Triage* is a French word meaning *to sort*. The goal is to do the greatest good for the greatest number of victims.

Finding Life-Threatened Victims

A variety of systems are used to identify care and transportation priorities. To find those needing immediate care for life-threatening conditions, first tell all victims who can get up and walk to move to a specific area. Victims who can get up and walk rarely have life-threatening injuries. These victims ("walking wounded") are classified as delayed priority (see below). Do not force a victim to move if he or she complains of pain.

Find the life-threatened victims by performing only the primary survey on all remaining victims. Go to motionless victims first. You must move rapidly (spend less than 60 seconds with each victim) from one victim to the next until all have been assessed. Classify victims according to the following care and transportation priorities:

1. *Immediate care.* Victim has life-threatening injuries but can be saved.
   - airway or breathing difficulties (not breathing or breathing rate faster than 30 per minute)
   - weak or no pulse
   - uncontrolled or severe bleeding
   - unresponsive or unconscious
2. *Urgent care.* Victims not fitting into the immediate or delayed categories. Care and transportation can be delayed up to one hour.
3. *Delayed care.* Victims with minor injuries. Care and transportation can be delayed up to three hours.
4. *Dead.* Victims are obviously dead, mortally wounded, or unlikely to survive because of the extent of their injuries, age, and medical condition.

Do not become involved in treating the victims at this point, but ask knowledgeable bystanders to care for immediate life-threatening problems (i.e., rescue breathing, bleeding control).

Reassess victims regularly for changes in their condition. Only when the immediate life-threatening conditions receive care should those with less serious conditions be given care.

Later, you will usually be relieved when more highly trained emergency personnel arrive on the scene. You may then be asked to provide first aid, to help move victims, or to help with ambulance or helicopter transportation.

Moving Victims

A victim should not be moved until he or she is ready for transportation to a hospital, if required. All necessary first aid should be provided first. A victim should be moved only if there is an immediate danger:

- There is a fire or danger of fire.
- Explosives or other hazardous materials are involved.

- It is impossible to protect the accident scene from hazards.
- It is impossible to gain access to other victims in the situation (e.g., a vehicle) who need life-saving care.

▼ CAUTION: DO NOT

- move a victim unless you absolutely have to. That might happen if the victim is in immediate danger or must be moved to shelter while waiting for the EMS to arrive.
- make the injury worse by moving the victim.
- move a victim who could have a spine injury.
- move a victim without stabilizing the injured part.
- move a victim unless you know where you are going.
- leave an unresponsive victim alone.
- move a victim when someone could be sent for help. Wait with the victim and send someone else for help.
- try to move a victim by yourself if other people are available to help.

A cardiac arrest victim is usually moved unless he or she is already on the ground or floor, because CPR must be performed on a firm surface.

Emergency Moves

The major danger in moving a victim quickly is the possibility of aggravating a spine injury. In an emergency, every effort should be made to pull the victim in the direction of the long axis of the body to provide as much protection to the spinal cord as possible. If victims are on the floor or ground, you can drag them away from the scene by one of various techniques.

Nonemergency Moves

All injured parts should be stabilized before and during moving. If rapid transportation is not needed, it is helpful to practice on another person about the same size as the injured victim.

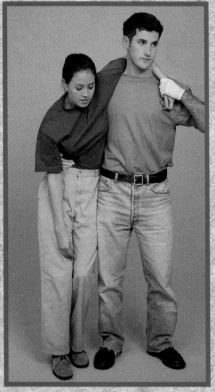

1.

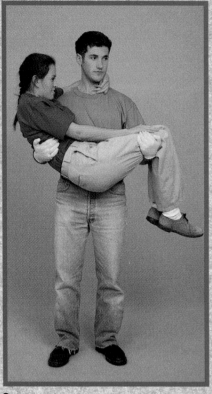

2.

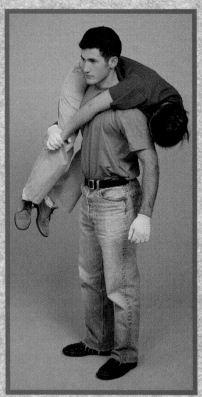

3.

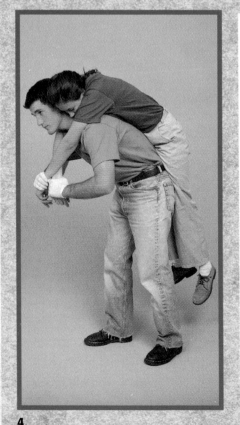

4.

1. *Human crutch* (*one person helps victim to walk*). If one leg is injured, help the victim to walk on the good leg while you support the injured side.

2. *Cradle carry.* Use for children and lightweight adults who cannot walk.

3. *Fireman's carry.* If the victim's injuries permit, longer distances can be traveled if the victim is carried over your shoulder.

4. *Pack-strap carry.* When injuries make the fireman's carry unsafe, this method is better for longer distances.

5. *Piggyback carry.* Use this method when the victim cannot walk but can use the arms to hang onto the rescuer.

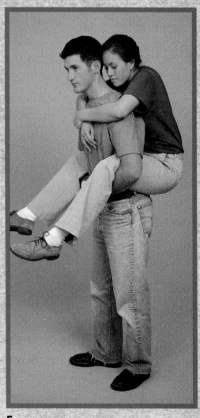

5.

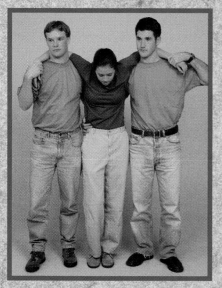

1.

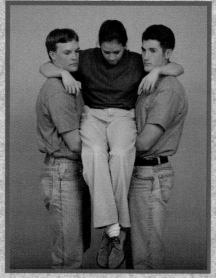

2.

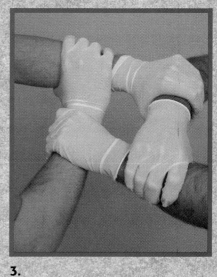

3.

1. *Two-person assist.* Similar to human crutch.
2. *Two-handed seat carry.*
3. *Four-handed seat carry.* The easiest two-person carry when no equipment is available, and the victim cannot walk but can use the arms to hang onto the two rescuers.
4. *Extremity carry.*
5. *Chair carry.* Useful for a narrow passage or up or down stairs. Use a sturdy chair that can take the victim's weight.
6. *Hammock carry.* Three to six people stand on alternate sides of the injured person and link hands beneath the victim.

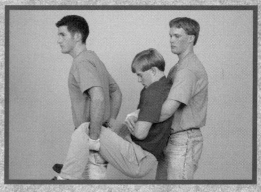

4.

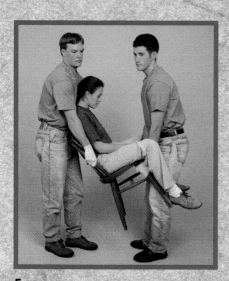

5.

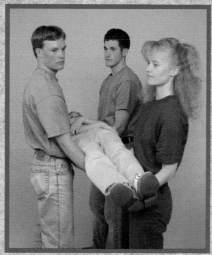

6.

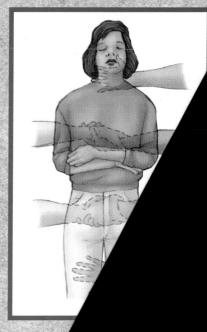

Quick Emergency Index

Moving Victims